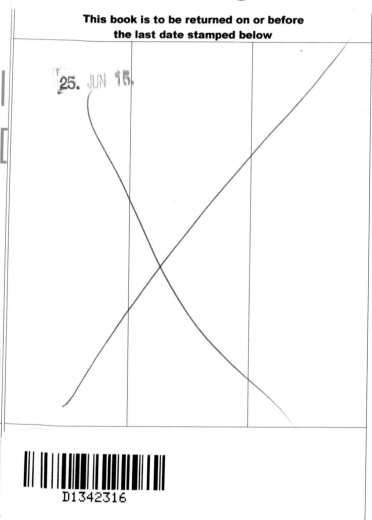

Also available from Remedica:

Anal and Rectal Diseases Explained
The IBD Yearbook Series
Pediatric Gastroenterology and Clinical Nutrition

View and purchase books at
www.remedicabooks.com

Published by Remedica
Commonwealth House, 1 New Oxford Street, London, WC1A 1NU, UK
Civic Opera Building, 20 North Wacker Drive, Suite 1642, Chicago, IL 60606, USA

info@remedicabooks.com
www.remedicabooks.com
Tel: +44 20 7759 2999
Fax: +44 20 7759 2901

Publisher: Andrew Ward
In-house editors: Catherine Booth and Carolyn Dunn
Design and artwork: AS&K Skylight Creative Services

Remedica is a member of the AS&K Media Partnership.

ISBN-13: 978 1 901346 56 5
ISBN-10: 1 901346 56 0

British Library Cataloguing-in-Publication Data
A catalogue record for this book is available from the British Library.

Immunology and Diseases of the Gut

Thomas T MacDonald, PhD, FRCPath, FMedSci
Professor of Immunology and Dean for Research
Barts and the London Queen Mary's School of Medicine and Dentistry
London
UK

Adrian C Bateman, BSc, MD, FRCPath
Consultant Histopathologist
Department of Cellular Pathology
Southampton General Hospital
Southampton
UK

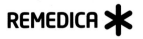

Author biographies

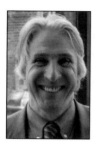

Professor Tom T MacDonald

Tom MacDonald is currently Professor of Immunology and Dean for Research at Barts and the London School of Medicine and Dentistry. His enthusiasm for gut immunology and inflammation was kindled by the late Professor Anne Ferguson, and after studying mouse gut immunology in the USA he returned to Bart's in the mid-1980s as a Wellcome Trust Senior Lecturer to work on gut inflammation in patients. He has over 300 publications on gut immunology and inflammation, including the first demonstrations that gluten elicits a T-cell cytokine response in celiac disease, activated Th1 cells cause the flat mucosa in the small bowel, Crohn's disease is a Th1-mediated disease, matrix metalloproteinases are mediators of gut ulcers, and that tumor necrosis factor is important in inflammatory bowel disease (IBD). His main current interest is the control of transforming growth factor-β signaling in IBD.

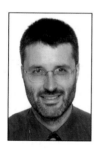

Dr Adrian C Bateman

Adrian Bateman was appointed as a Consultant Histopathologist to Southampton General Hospital in 1997 after initial qualification in medicine at the Charing Cross and Westminster Medical School. He specializes in gastrointestinal pathology and, in this role, has a close working relationship with members of the clinical teams responsible for the management of gastrointestinal disease in Southampton. His research interests include the role of the immune system in disease pathogenesis and progression.

Preface

The gut is the interface between the tissues and the external environment, covered for most of its length by only a single layer of epithelium. The need for adequate host defence against infections in the gut means that the body must make a major investment in populating the gut with lymph nodes and immune cells. At the same time, the gut immune system, by over-reacting to harmless foods or gut microbes, is also responsible for causing gut disease. New treatments for gut inflammation in patients are primarily based on manipulating the immune response.

While it may seem self-evident to an immunologist that, to understand gut diseases with an inflammatory/immunological component, an understanding of immunology is a prerequisite, this is largely not the case in the histopathology and gastroenterology community. The blame for this lies squarely with immunologists themselves, who delight in acronyms and complexity and who have failed to relate their discipline to gut diseases. Look in any textbook of immunology and you will see only a small section devoted to gut immunology and nothing on gut inflammation or gut disease. Immunology does not figure highly in the curriculum at most medical schools, so students graduate with only a haphazard understanding, if any understanding at all.

The purpose of this book, therefore, is to attempt to remedy this situation and to provide a life line. We have tried to explain immunology at the most basic level needed to understand gut diseases. For example, it is impossible to understand celiac disease without knowing something about human leukocyte antigen, or Crohn's disease without knowing about T-helper 1 cells. For ease of reference, we have listed gut diseases alphabetically, and, wherever possible, tied the disease to the immunology. Professor Thomas T. MacDonald is delighted to have been joined in this effort by Dr Adrian C. Bateman, a consultant histopathologist with an interest in the gut.

Thomas T. MacDonald
Adrian C. Bateman
June 2006

Acknowledgments

The authors wish to thank the following colleagues who helped by providing slides: Prof. Martin Zeitz, Prof. Paola Domizio, Prof. Neil Shepherd, Dr Bryan Warren, Prof. Per Brandtzaeg, Dr Jo Spencer, Dr Alan Phillips, Prof. Marco Novelli, Dr Sylvia Pender, Dr Art Anderson, Dr Tim Stephenson, and Dr Robert Owen.

Contents

Glossary

Index

Abbreviations

AA	amyloid-associated protein
APC	antigen-presenting cell
ASCA	antibodies to *Saccharomyces cerevisiae*
C region	constant region
CARD	caspase activation and recruitment domain
CD	cluster of differentiation
CGD	chronic granulomatous disease
CMI	cell-mediated immunity
CRP	C-reactive protein
CTLA	cytotoxic T-lymphocyte antigen
D region	diversity region
DCC	deleted in colorectal carcinoma
EATL	enteropathy-associated T-cell lymphoma
EBV	Epstein–Barr virus
ELISA	enzyme-linked immunoabsorbent assay
ER	endoplasmic reticulum
FAE	follicle-associated epithelium
FAP	familial adenomatous polyposis
GC	germinal center
GVHD	graft-versus-host disease
HEV	high endothelial venule
HLA	human leukocyte antigen
HNPCC	hereditary nonpolyposis colorectal cancer
IBD	inflammatory bowel disease
ICAM	intercellular cell adhesion molecule
IEL	intraepithelial lymphocyte
IFN	interferon
Ig	immunoglobulin
IL	interleukin
J region	joining region
LFA	lymphocyte function-associated antigen
LP	lamina propria
LPS	lipopolysaccharide
M cell	microfold cell
MAdCAM	mucosal addressin cell adhesion molecule
MHC	major histocompatibility complex

MMP	matrix metalloproteinase
NEC	neonatal necrotizing enterocolitis
NOD	nucleotide-binding oligomerization domain
NSAID	non-steroidal anti-inflammatory drug
PAF	platelet-activating factor
PAS	periodic acid-Schiff
PP	Peyer's patch
PTLD	post-transplant lymphoproliferative disorder
RAG	recombination-activating gene
SCID	severe combined immunodeficiency
TAP	transporter of antigenic peptides
TB	tuberculosis
TCR	T-cell receptor
TdT	terminal deoxyribonucleotidyl transferase
Th1	T-helper cell type I
Th2	T-helper cell type II
TIMP	tissue inhibitor of metalloproteinase
TLR	Toll-like receptor
TNF	tumor necrosis factor
tTG	tissue transglutaminase
UC	ulcerative colitis
V region	variable region
VacA	vacuolating toxin A

1 A Beginner's Guide to Immunology

Introduction

Immunology is very complicated. There are myriad different cells and molecules that interact with one another in a seemingly bewildering fashion. For this reason, many people find the subject intimidating. Nonetheless, many diseases that affect the gut are immune mediated. In other words, the main problem is the immune system itself – usually overreacting to something within the intestine. To fully understand these diseases, then, you must grasp some indispensable aspects of basic immunology.

Overview

The purpose of the immune system is to protect the tissues and fluids of the body from infection. Many microorganisms have evolved to live and multiply in our tissues, and they have many strategies by which to enter the body. For example: the malaria parasite is injected into the body in the proboscis of a mosquito as it penetrates the epidermis to feed on blood; some bacteria, such as *Vibrio cholerae*, do not even enter the tissues of the body, but colonize the surface of the gut; and soil microbes can enter any tissue through traumatic injury. Consequently, the cells of the immune system, which arise from stem cells in the bone marrow, must constantly patrol the tissues to combat these invaders.

Innate immunity
(the non-specific immune response)

If bacteria enter the skin through a cut, or invade the gut wall, the initial response involves non-specific inflammatory cells. Tissue macrophages in the skin have cell-surface receptors – the Toll-like receptors (TLRs) – that bind various bacterial

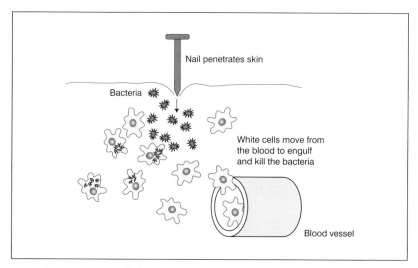

Figure 1. In the non-specific immune response, the body mobilizes phagocytic white cells to move from the blood into the tissues. These then engulf and kill the invading bacteria. In this example, the bacteria have been carried into the skin on a rusty nail.

components. TLR9, for example, specifically recognizes bacterial DNA, TLR5 recognizes bacterial flagellin, and TLR4 recognizes lipopolysaccharide (LPS), a major component of the Gram-negative bacterial cell wall.

The binding of these components to the appropriate TLR tells the macrophage to produce proinflammatory cytokines, such as tumor necrosis factor (TNF)α and interleukin (IL)-1β. These then tell the endothelial cells lining the blood vessels to increase their expression of adhesion molecules, and to capture onto their surface passing white blood cells (neutrophils and macrophages). These white cells migrate across the blood vessel wall into the tissue where they attempt to engulf and kill the bacteria (**Figure 1**). If this is successful then the infection is cleared.

Bacteria, however, have evolved many strategies to avoid being killed by the host cells, and may even divide faster than the host cells can kill them. If this is the case then persistent infection occurs. Organisms that leak into the blood are potentially very dangerous (causing septicemia), so the liver and spleen are also full of macrophages that can kill the microorganisms as the blood passes through these tissues.

The importance of this type of innate immunity is illustrated in children with chronic granulomatous disease (CGD), who have a defect in one of the enzyme pathways that white cells use to kill bacteria. These children suffer from infections that cause chronic draining abscesses, full of pus. Microabscesses form in the gut of CGD children because normal gut bacteria that are usually killed by phagocytes after crossing the epithelium are not killed and persist. Interestingly, some children develop gut inflammation like Crohn's disease.

Adaptive immunity (the specific immune response)

Because innate immunity is not complete, the immune system can also call upon the specific (or adaptive) arm of the immune response. In this type of response, lymphocytes (T and B cells, described below) specifically recognize parts of an infectious agent (antigens) and activate many different pathways to eliminate it. One of the main ways that T cells do this is by secreting cytokines, which make neutrophils and macrophages much more efficient at killing bacteria. For a definition of an antigen, see **Box 1**.

For the specific arm of the immune response to be activated, lymphocytes have to recognize and respond to microorganisms in the lymph nodes. Microorganisms are carried into the nodes in lymph: small lymphatic vessels in the skin drain into larger vessels, which enter the lymph nodes. These lymph nodes are strategically scattered throughout the body (**Figure 2**). Amongst the dozens of lymph nodes in the body are:

- the submandibular lymph nodes in the neck, which deal with infections around the mouth and throat
- the inguinal lymph nodes in the groin, which deal with infections in the legs
- the axillary lymph nodes in the armpits, which deal with infections in the arms

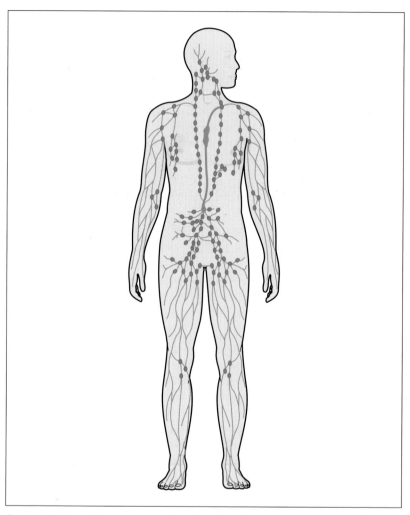

Figure 2. The lymphatic drainage and lymph nodes of the body. Lymph nodes in the gut are not shown. A network of vessels drains the tissue fluids of the extremities and passes into the lymph nodes in the groin, armpits, and neck, and along the spine.

Once the microorganism has entered the lymph nodes, specific lymphocytes respond to its presence. Lymphocytes (T cells, in particular) also patrol the body looking for infectious microorganisms. As blood flows through a lymph node, lymphocytes adhere to a specialized blood vessel (the high endothelial venule [HEV]) and crawl across the vessel wall into the node itself (**Figure 3**). If a lymphocyte does not recognize its specific antigen then it enters the efferent lymphatic, which leaves the lymph node and drains via the thoracic duct into

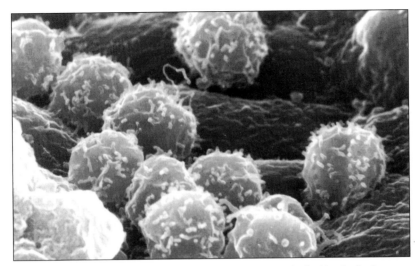

Figure 3. Scanning electron microscope image of lymphocytes in the blood adhering to the surface of the high endothelial venule.
Magnification ×1,000.

the blood, where the process starts again. This is called lymphocyte recirculation, and each lymphocyte goes through this cycle every 24–48 hours. Activated lymphocytes also leave blood vessels in tissues such as the skin or lungs. These drain back into the lymph nodes via afferent lymphatics, and then back into the blood via efferent lymphatics.

The gut is the most vulnerable site of the human body, so there are abundant lymph nodes from the mouth to the anus; the tonsils are located in the back of the throat; the small intestine contains hundreds of special lymph nodes called Peyer's patches (PP) (see **Chapter 2**); there is the appendix in the cecum and thousands of small lymph nodes (follicles) throughout the colon wall. The small intestine also contains many thousands of these isolated lymphoid follicles. In all, 85% of the body's lymph nodes are in the gut.

Antigen recognition

Infectious agents that enter the lymph nodes trigger specific immune responses. But how do the cells of the immune system recognize these agents, and how can they possibly recognize millions of different foreign molecules (antigens) that the body has not previously been exposed to? The answer lies in genes on chromosomes 2, 14, and 22, which encode protein cell surface receptors on

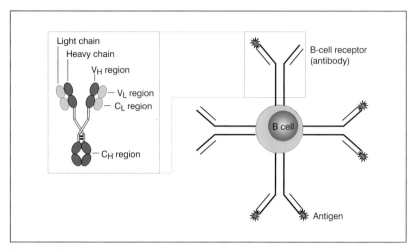

Figure 4. Diagrammatic illustration of an antibody molecule on a B cell. B cells have several hundred-thousand antibody molecules anchored on their surface. Through these they recognize a specific foreign antigen. In virgin B cells that are freshly emerged from the bone marrow, these cell-surface antibody molecules are IgM and IgD, which have identical V domains. When activated, B cells secrete additional antibodies with the same V domain as the cell-surface antibody. C: constant; Ig: immunoglobulin; V: variable.

B cells, and genes on chromosomes 7 and 14, which encode protein cell surface receptors on T cells. T and B cells are covered in receptors that recognize foreign antigens; but individual T and B cells only recognize a single antigen.

B cells

The surface membrane of a newly formed B cell in the bone marrow contains several hundred-thousand B-cell receptors. These receptors are antibody molecules (**Figure 4**), all of which recognize the same antigen.

- Each antibody is made up of two **heavy** chains and two **light** chains. Heavy chains come in five types (μ, δ, γ, ϵ, α), while light chains come in two types (κ and λ). On a single B cell, each antibody has two identical heavy chains and two identical light chains.
- Each heavy-chain and light-chain has a **constant** (C) part of the molecule.
- Each heavy-chain and light chain has a **variable** (V) part of the molecule.
- In heavy and light chains, part of the molecule is also encoded by **joining** (J) region genes. This part is found between the C and V region.
- Heavy chains also contain a **diversity** (D) region, encoded by D-region genes, which are inserted between the V- and J-region genes (**Figure 5**).

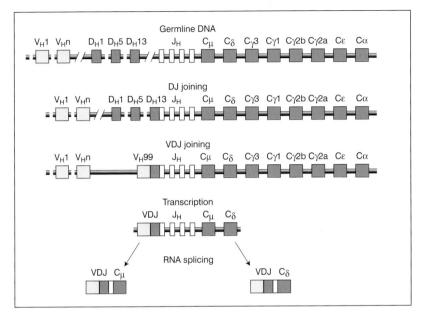

Figure 5. The mechanism by which many different antibody specificities can be made by mixing and matching different gene segments. The example shown illustrates how a single B cell makes IgM and IgD molecules, which then function as cell-surface antigen receptors. There are multiple variable (V), diversity (D), and joining (J) genes, but only a single copy of the different heavy (H)-chain constant (C) domain genes. The first part of the rearrangement involves "looping out" a piece of DNA between D and J to bring the D and J genes together. In the next step, more DNA is looped out to bring a V gene next to the combined DJ genes (VDJ joining). RNA is then made of VDJ and C_μ and C_δ, which, by RNA splicing, makes RNA with VDJ and C_μ, and a separate RNA with VDJ and C_δ. Each is then translated into protein and inserted into the cell membrane. Ig: immunoglobulin.

Gene shuffling

The key to our ability to make millions of different antibody molecules – so that we can recognize any pathogen we meet – lies in the many genes that encode the V, D, and J domains of each antibody molecule. By shuffling these genes, it is possible to make tens of millions of different antibody molecules.

For example, for λ chains there are three functional V genes and three functional J genes, and for κ chains there are 350 functional V genes and four functional J genes. During B-cell development, these genes are rearranged so that a single V gene is put next to a single J gene and a single C gene. This makes up a cluster of genes that encodes a single light-chain protein. Because each individual gene encodes a protein of a slightly different shape, each VJC recombination produces a protein of a different shape. Simple mathematics tells us that random rearrangement of VJ genes can produce nine different λ-chain proteins and 1,400 different κ-chain proteins.

For heavy chains, the story is made slightly more complex by the presence of D genes, but the principle is the same. In mice, for example, there are several hundred heavy-chain V genes, 30 D genes, and six J genes – by recombination, these can give rise to 36,000 different heavy-chain proteins.

A process called **allelic exclusion** means that a single B cell makes only one type of heavy chain and one type of light chain: once recombination occurs on one chromosome, allelic exclusion prevents recombination from occurring on the other chromosome (we each have one set of chromosomes from our mother and one from our father).

When the cell makes an antibody it combines two heavy chains and two light chains. If a µ heavy chain is combined with a κ light chain then it is easy to see that it is possible to make 50 million different µκ combinations. The V, D, and J genes encode for different polypeptides; therefore, each of these 50 million different antibodies (and therefore potentially 50 million different B cells) has cell-surface proteins of a different shape, into which can fit 50 million different antigens (**Figure 6**).

Other mechanisms

Finally, there are mechanisms by which the potential number of antibodies made can be expanded further (ie, N-region insertions). As a B cell is rearranging its V, D, and J heavy-chain genes, an enzyme called terminal deoxyribonucleotidyl transferase (TdT) randomly inserts DNA bases at the cut ends as the recombination occurs. If TdT inserts three bases that encode for an amino acid such as lysine, then when the antibody molecule is made it will have an additional lysine in its V domain. This will slightly change its shape so that it can bind different antigens.

T cells

T cell precursors come from the bone marrow and mature T-cell development occurs in the thymus. T cells also recognize antigens using specific cell-surface receptors. There are two types of T-cell receptors (TCRs), each of which is made up of two transmembrane polypeptide chains, which are linked with a disulfide bond.

Most T cells express the αβ form of the TCR – ie, the receptor is made of a single α chain and a single β chain, joined together. A minority of T cells in the body express the γδ receptor – ie, the receptor is made of a single γ chain and a single δ chain. Cells expressing the γδ receptor are particularly abundant in the gut epithelium.

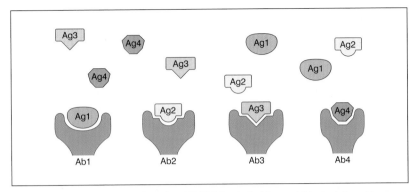

Figure 6. The consequence of random VDJ joining is that the variable domains of heavy and light chains on the antibody molecule make up a shape into which an antigen can fit. Since it is possible to make millions of different antibodies from DNA, B cells can recognize millions of different antigens. In this figure, antibody variable domains (of which there are two on each antibody), made up of V_H and V_L, make molecules with different shapes (Ab1–n) that bind different-shaped antigens (Ag1–n).

Gene shuffling

As in B cells, each chain in T cells (α, β, γ, or δ) has a C domain (ie, a part of the molecule that remains the same between different T cells and different individuals) and a V domain (which is different between different T cells). Some chains also have D and J domains. There are around 50 Vα genes and 70 Jα genes, so that it is possible to make 3,500 different α chains. The β-chain locus contains 57 Vβ genes, two Dβ genes, and 13 Jβ genes, which can encode for almost 1,500 different β chains. Again, simple mathematics says that germline α and β genes can encode about 5 million different $\alpha\beta$ TCRs.

The γ chain has 14 Vγ genes and five Jγ genes, and the δ locus has three Vδ genes, three Dδ genes, and three Jδ genes. These can therefore also encode multiple receptors.

Other mechanisms

Again, TdT can also add bases to all rearranging α, β, γ, and δ chains, dramatically increasing the number of different TCRs that can be made.

An interesting feature of T cells is that, while allelic exclusion occurs in the β chain of the TCR, it does not occur in the α chain. Consequently, T cells can have two different TCRs on their membrane with a common β chain, coupled to rearranged α chains for each allele. Thus, strictly speaking, individual T cells can have two different specificities.

How do T and B cells recognize foreign antigens, ie, non-self and not self-antigens?

Because T and B cells with millions of different receptors are randomly produced, some of these receptors will be able to recognize and bind to self proteins/peptides, since there is no way that this can be predicted. Consequently, T and B cells are "censored" before they are allowed to move into the peripheral lymphoid organs. A breakdown in this system can result in autoimmune disease.

B cells

Censoring of B cells occurs in two ways. Firstly, if a new B cell is made in the bone marrow from a lymphoid stem cell and its cell-surface receptors bind to an antigen that is present locally, perhaps from the blood, then the cell undergoes apoptosis (ie, kills itself). Alternatively, the cell might be made anergic (ie, unresponsive). This is potentially dangerous because anergic B cells are still alive and autoimmune disease can occur if the anergy is overcome. Mature B cells then migrate to the lymphoid organs.

T cells

T cells are so-called because they come from the thymus: a creamish, bi-lobed tissue that is located just above the heart in the chest cavity. The thymus is large in neonates and children, but after adolescence it involutes and becomes infiltrated with fat. Essentially, the thymus has done its work by birth; neonatal removal of the thymus (as often occurs during cardiac surgery) has no effect on T-cell immunity. T-cell precursors leave the marrow and enter the blood. They then cross into the outermost region of the thymus, the cortex, where they undergo rapid division, giving rise to thousands of daughter cells. Most of these cells die *in situ*. The reasons for this are now understood.

Unlike B cells, T cells only recognize peptide fragments of antigens presented by major histocompatibility complex (MHC) molecules on the surface of antigen-presenting cells (APCs) (see below). If, in the thymus, a T cell is made whose TCR binds strongly to a self peptide on an MHC molecule then the T cell undergoes apoptosis (**Figure 7**). This is called **negative selection** or **clonal deletion** and is a mechanism to stop T-cell autoimmunity. If the TCR does not bind to any peptide on an MHC molecule in the thymus then the T cell also undergoes apoptosis. This is called **death by neglect**.

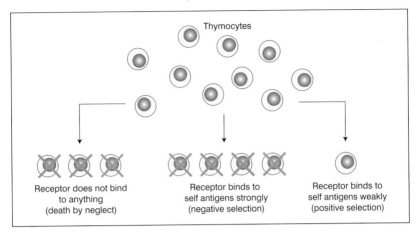

Figure 7. In the thymus, especially early in our lives, there is rearrangement of TCR genes to produce T cells with the potential to recognize millions of different antigens. Since this process is random, many T cells that recognize self antigens are produced. There has to be vigorous censoring of these T cells to avoid autoimmune disease. Consequently, those T cells whose receptors bind strongly to self antigens are destroyed in the thymus (clonal deletion). T cells whose receptors do not bind to anything in the thymus also die (death by neglect). Only those T cells that bind weakly to self antigens in the thymus are allowed to mature and leave the thymus (positive selection). They bind so weakly to self antigens that they will not be triggered in the periphery and cause autoimmune disease. Once in the lymphoid tissue, there is a random chance that a T cell will recognize an MHC molecule that presents a peptide from a pathogen. If so, this complex will bind with high affinity to the TCR, starting a cascade of events that leads to T-cell activation. MHC: major histocompatibility complex; TCR: T-cell receptor.

If, however, the TCR binds weakly to a peptide on an MHC molecule then the T cell receives a positive signal, it matures, and enters the thymic medulla. This is called **positive selection**. The need to cull self-reactive or non-reactive T cells is very stringent, and 99.9% of T cells never actually leave the thymus, but die *in situ*.

From the medulla, T cells enter the blood and eventually reach the lymphoid tissue. Once in the lymphoid tissue, there is a random chance that a T cell will recognize an MHC molecule that presents a peptide from a pathogen. If so, this complex will bind with high affinity to the TCR, starting a cascade of events that leads to T-cell activation.

Antigen presentation

B cells

The presentation of antigens to B cells is very simple: B-cell receptors are antibodies (usually immunologbulin [Ig]M), which can directly bind foreign proteins, lipids, and carbohydrate antigens. Cross-linking of the receptors delivers a signal to the B cell to start to divide and make daughter cells, which make antibodies. These antibodies are also IgM – exactly the same molecule as the IgM on the surface that functioned as a receptor. For the cell to make IgG, IgA, and IgE, however, it requires T-cell help (see below).

T cells

For T cells, antigen presentation is more complex. T cells recognize fragments of foreign antigens, usually short peptides of 8–20 amino acids long. The situation is further complicated because TCRs can only recognize the peptides when they are bound to, or presented on, surface molecules on APCs. These surface molecules are encoded by the MHC (in humans, the human leukocyte antigen [HLA] gene system) (**Figure 8** and **Box 2**).

MHC molecules

MHC molecules come in two main types: class I and class II. MHC class I molecules are present on all cells except red cells, and are made up of a single heavy chain and a light chain (β_2-microglobulin). MHC class II molecules are usually found on APCs and are made up of two transmembrane chains: α and β. APCs are usually dendritic cells and macrophages, but B cells are also efficient APCs, especially to memory T cells (see **Glossary**).

MHC molecules vary hugely between individuals, which is why it is difficult to match recipients and donors for organ transplantation. At the region of the molecule furthest away from the cell membrane, MHC molecules have a cleft or groove that can bind short peptides for presentation to T cells. The variability between MHC molecules largely occurs in this region.

Antigen presentation to T cells

There are two main populations of T cells in the body: those that express CD4 and those that express CD8. These cells have different functions and recognize different MHC molecules. CD4 cells recognize peptides bound to MHC class II molecules on the surface of APCs, while CD8 cells recognize peptides bound to MHC class I molecules.

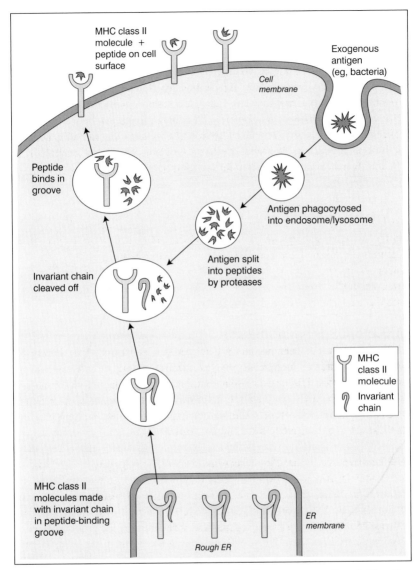

Figure 8. MHC class II molecule antigen presentation (the exogenous pathway). Class II molecules are made in the rough ER, where their peptide-binding groove is masked by invariant chain. Invariant chain is cleaved off as the molecule moves to the cell surface, which allows peptides from phagocytosed antigen to bind to the MHC class II molecule. On the surface, the foreign peptide can then be recognized by T cells.
ER: endoplasmic reticulum; MHC: major histocompatibility complex.

MHC class II presentation to CD4 T cells

This is called the **exogenous pathway** of antigen processing (see **Figure 8**). Through this pathway, foreign antigens (ie, proteins, viruses, or bacteria) that are outside the cell are eliminated. APCs phagocytose the antigen into a structure in the cell called an endosome. The internalized antigen then passes into a structure called a lysosome. Endosomes and lysosomes are acidic and contain enzymes that break the antigen into short peptides. In the cytoplasm, the endosome/lysosome then fuses with vesicles containing MHC class II molecules that have been synthesized in the Golgi body.

Importantly, when MHC class II molecules are made in the endoplasmic reticulum (ER) their peptide-binding groove is occupied by a molecule called **invariant chain**, which prevents self peptides from entering the groove. Invariant chain is cleaved off when the vesicle containing the newly made MHC class II molecules fuses with the lysosome containing the exogenous peptides. Those peptides that fit in the groove are then sent to the cell surface, where they can be seen by a T cell as a combination of non-self peptide and self MHC molecule. If a T cell has a receptor specific for this combination, then it is activated.

MHC class I presentation to CD8 cells

This is called the **endogenous pathway** of antigen presentation (**Figure 9**). Through this pathway, antigens that are present inside cells (eg, those from

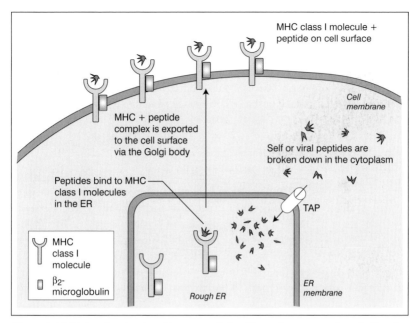

Figure 9. MHC class I molecule antigen presentation (the endogenous pathway). Class I molecules are made in the rough ER. A special peptide pump, TAP, delivers peptides from the cytoplasm into the ER, where they bind to class I molecules and are sent, via the Golgi body, to the cell surface. Class I molecules are present on all cell surfaces except for those of red blood cells, and the peptide-binding groove is occupied by self peptides. This is how the immune system can become tolerant to antigens inside cells, since, in the thymus, a T cell that bound well to a self peptide on a class I molecule would be deleted. During viral infection, viral peptides transported into the ER displace the self peptides from class I molecules and are transported to the surface of the cell, where they can be recognized by T cells. ER: endoplasmic reticulum; MHC: major histocompatibility complex; TAP: transporter of antigenic peptides.

viruses) are eliminated. MHC class I molecules also have a peptide-binding groove. When class I molecules are made, they are passed into the rough ER. The membrane of the ER contains special pumps (transporter of antigenic peptides [TAP]) whose function is to pass any peptide (both self peptides and foreign antigens) from the cytoplasm of the cell into the ER.

There is constant transport of peptides produced by degradation of self molecules into the ER. If a virus infects the cell, viral peptides are also transported into the ER by TAP molecules. If these peptides bind to the peptide-binding groove of the MHC molecule then they are exported to the cell surface (via the Golgi body), where they can be seen by T cells.

In healthy people, MHC class I molecules on cell surfaces are occupied by self peptides. It is the body's way of knowing what antigens are inside cells and, of course, in the thymus, self peptides are presented to newly-made T cells on MHC class I molecules and self-reactive CD8 cells are killed. During a viral infection, viral peptides transported into the ER will replace self peptides and be transported to the surface of the cell, where they can be seen by T cells.

T-cell activation

Binding to a peptide/MHC complex is the initial and most crucial event in T-cell activation, and controls the specificity of cell-mediated immunity (CMI). However, it is insufficient for the cell to simply divide and become activated. The TCR is associated with a cluster of proteins called the CD3 complex. All T cells express CD3, which makes it a very useful marker for T cells in blood and tissues. When peptide-binding occurs, the CD3 complex passes a signal to the nucleus to begin activation. T cells, however, need to be activated by signals from other molecules on APC.

In CD4 T cells, the CD4 molecule itself binds to an MHC class II molecule and then activates parts of the CD3 complex. In CD8 cells, the CD8 molecule binds to an MHC class I molecule and activates the same process. In addition, an array of other molecules on the T cell and APC come together to bind the T cell closely to the APC and deliver activation signals. Some can even deliver negative signals and switch the T cell off.

The best characterized of these are the CD80/CD86 molecules on APC. If they bind to CD28 on T cells then an activation signal is delivered. If, however, they bind to cytotoxic T-lymphocyte antigen (CTLA)4 on T cells, the cell switches off. CD28-knockout mice have impaired T-cell function, while CTLA4-knockout mice have very enhanced T-cell function, and die of autoimmune disease. Another molecule on T cells, CD40L, binds to CD40 on APC and delivers an accessory activation signal. Yet another example is lymphocyte function-associated antigen (LFA)1 on T cells, which binds to intercellular cell adhesion molecule (ICAM)1 on APC. Likewise, CD2 on T cells binds to LFA3 on APC.

Collectively, these are called **accessory molecules**. Generally, the function of accessory molecules appears to be to regulate the magnitude and type of response following T-cell recognition of foreign peptides. **Figure 10** illustrates some of the molecules associated with the TCR.

A Beginner's Guide to Immunology

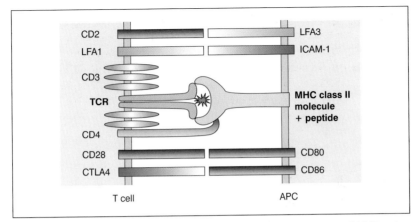

Figure 10. T-cell activation requires much more than simple recognition of self MHC and peptide. The TCR confers the specificity of the response, but a T cell will not become activated unless a number of other interactions occur between the T cell and the APC. These include CD4 binding to MHC class II molecules (or CD8 binding to MHC class I molecules), CD2 to LFA3, LFA1 to ICAM-1, CD28 to CD80, and CTLA4 to CD86. All of these interactions signal to the T cell that it needs to respond. APC: antigen-presenting cell; CTLA: cytotoxic T-lymphocyte antigen; ICAM: intercellular cell adhesion molecule; LFA: lymphocyte function-associated antigen; MHC: major histocompatibility complex; TCR: T-cell receptor.

T-cell function

Once all of these interactions have taken place, the T cell undergoes rapid division. Since all of the daughter cells are the same, this process is called **clonal expansion**. T cells produce a molecule, IL-2, which feeds back to bind to a specific receptor on the same T cell and drives this expansion **(Figure 11)**. In the case of viral infections, up to 60% of the cells in the blood may be virus specific.

CD4 T cells and CD8 T cells have different functions **(Figure 12)**. CD4 cells help B cells and regulate CMI. They also make interferon (IFN)γ and TNFα, which not only make cells resistant to further infections, but also activate macrophages to phagocytose viruses and bacteria **(Figure 13)**. CD8 cells expand and become cytotoxic cells, and will kill cells that express the same peptide/MHC class I combination as originally led to their activation.

CD4 T cells differentiate along at least two pathways **(Figure 14)**: they can become T-helper cell type I (Th1) cells or T-helper cell type II (Th2) cells.

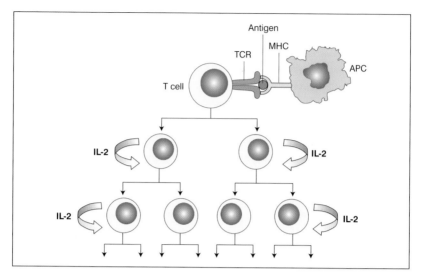

Figure 11. Clonal expansion of T cells and B cells is the hallmark of the immune response. Since we need to make T and B cells that recognize millions of different antigens, it follows that, in each of us, only a few individual T or B cells will recognize a given antigen. It is therefore important that these few cells divide rapidly to combat an infection. For T cells, expansion is dependent on IL-2. Made by activated T cells, IL-2 binds to the IL-2 receptor on T cells and causes T cells to divide. Indeed, IL-2 was originally called "T-cell growth factor". The cytotoxic drugs and irradiation that are used in cancer treatment stop T cells from dividing and undergoing clonal expansion, which is why these treatments also cause immune suppression. APC: antigen-presenting cell; IL: interleukin; MHC: major histocompatibility complex; TCR: T-cell receptor.

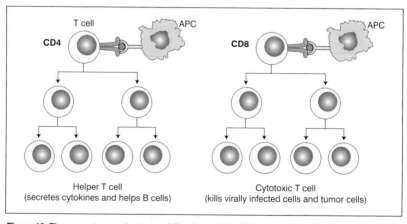

Figure 12. There are two main types of T cells, which differentiate from a CD4+CD8+ precursor in the thymus. CD4 cells recognize antigens presented on MHC class II molecules, secrete cytokines, and help B cells to make antibodies. CD8 cells recognize antigens presented on MHC class I molecules, and differentiate into cytotoxic T cells. APC: antigen-presenting cell; MHC: major histocompatibility complex.

A Beginner's Guide to Immunology

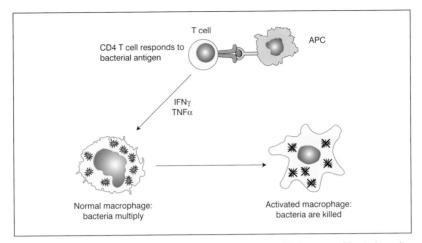

Figure 13. The mechanism of CD4 T-cell mediated immunity. Many types of bacteria and viruses can live and multiply in macrophages. T-cell-derived IFNγ and TNFα, however, can activate macrophages and increase their ability to kill viruses and bacteria. APC: antigen-presenting cell; IFN: interferon; TNF: tumor necrosis factor.

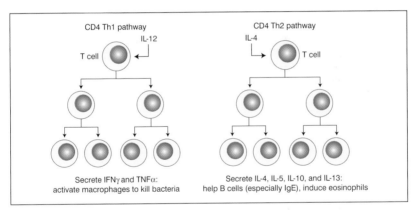

Figure 14. There are two types of CD4 cells. Th1 cells secrete IFNγ and TNFα and are important in cell-mediated immunity and delayed-type hypersensitivity (see **Chapter 3**). IL-12, which is made by macrophages, drives T cells along this pathway. Th2 cells make cytokines such as IL-4, IL-5, IL-10, and IL-13. These cytokines bind to B cells and drive them to become IgG-, IgA-, and IgE-producing plasma cells. Th2 cells differentiate along this pathway under the influence of IL-4, in this case made by mast cells. Excess production of IL-4 drives IgE responses, which cause allergies. IFN: interferon; Ig: immunoglobulin; IL: interleukin; Th: T-helper cell; TNF: tumor necrosis factor.

The Th1 pathway

APCs produce IL-12 when they encounter bacteria or bacterially derived molecules that activate TLRs. When a T cell recognises an antigen in the presence of IL-12, it becomes a Th1 cell. Th1 cells secrete IFNγ and TNFα, which activate macrophages and allow them to kill bacteria both inside and outside the cell (see **Figure 13**). Unfortunately, when too much IFNγ or TNFα is produced, the macrophages start killing normal cells and damaging tissues. Activated macrophages themselves make TNFα, IL-1, and IL-6, all of which cause injury when produced in excess. Crohn's disease is an example of a gut disease where T cells reacting to the bacterial flora in the gut activate macrophages in the gut wall to make excess amounts of TNFα.

The Th2 pathway

If a CD4 T cell encounters a peptide/MHC combination in the presence of IL-4 (from mast cells), it proceeds along the Th2 pathway. Th2 cells produce quite different cytokines: they make IL-4, IL-5, IL-10, and IL-13, all of which bind to B cells and drive them to become IgG-, IgA-, and IgE-producing plasma cells (**Figure 15**). This is why antibody responses are T-cell dependent, and, indeed, why CD4 cells were originally called T-helper cells. In some individuals, Th2 cells make too much IL-4, which drives IgE responses and results in allergies (see **Chapter 3**).

Antibody function

B cells can differentiate into plasma cells (antibody-producing factories) by 4–5 days after immunization. These can secrete antibodies into the serum, or into secretions that can bind to and help neutralize infections. These are **polyclonal antibodies** (**Box 3**). Plasma cells can make IgM, IgG, IgA, or IgE. IgM is the first antibody made, while the other classes are made by a process called **isotype switching**. This involves splicing V-domain genes onto different heavy-chain genes within daughter cells in the germinal centers (GCs) of the spleen and lymph nodes. In addition, the ability of B cells to make antibodies that bind very tightly to antigens is enhanced by a process called **somatic hypermutation** (see **Glossary**), which occurs in the GCs of the spleen and lymph nodes.

Some examples

The specificity of an antibody is conferred by its V domain, but its function is controlled by its C domain. Here are a few examples of the various functions of antibodies.

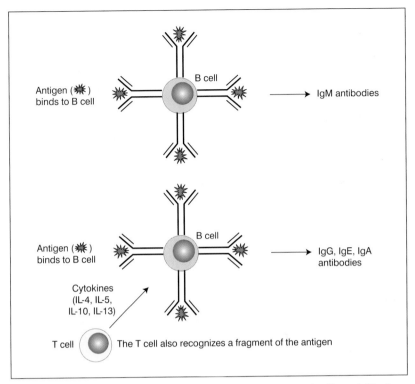

Figure 15. The concept of T-cell help. The antibody response to most antigens is T-cell dependent. When antigens bind to B cells directly, they stimulate IgM antibodies to be produced. However, in order for that B cell to continue to divide and go on to make IgG, IgE, and IgA antibodies it needs T-cell help. The T cells recognize peptides from the same antigen as the B cell and secrete cytokines such as IL-4, IL-5, IL-6, and IL-13, which are potent B-cell growth and differentiation factors. The process by which B cells first make IgM and then IgG, IgE, or IgA is called class or isotype switching. Ig: immunoglobulin; IL: interleukin.

IgM

Is very good at activating the complement cascade. This is a process by which antibody molecules binding to cells or bacteria initiate the activation of serum complement components, to assemble a macromolecular complex that can punch holes in cell membranes or bacteria. (**Figure 16**).

IgG

Has a number of different subclasses: IgG1, IgG2, and IgG3 also activate the complement cascade, but IgG4 does not. A major feature of complement activation is that fragments of complement are activated and released during the cascade. Some of these, such as C3a and C5a, are chemotactic for neutrophils

Box 3. Antibodies

Polyclonal antibodies

* When you inject a complex protein antigen into an animal, the animal makes serum antibodies.
* Because different B cells bind to different parts of the protein, many different B-cell clones are activated. These give rise to different plasma cells, making antibodies to different parts of the antigen.
* Hence, serum antibodies are polyclonal.
* These are useful, but polyclonal antibodies may cross-react and require live animals that have to be periodically bled.

Monoclonal antibodies

* In this technique, individual B cells are fused to make antibodies with tumor cells.
* The fused cell (hybridoma) continues to grow because it is a cancer cell, and secretes antibodies because it is a B cell.
* Because you can clone a single hybridoma cell, it is possible to make antibodies of a single specificity and to make them in large amounts *in vitro*.
* Monoclonal antibody production is hit and miss and requires a lot of screening.

Example
* Inject a mouse with human T cells and it makes antibodies to everything that is different between its own T cells and human T cells.
* Make hybridomas and clone out individual cells (maybe 300–500 clones).
* Screen the supernatants of these clones for antibodies that bind to human T cells, but not to B cells, macrophages, mast cells, etc.
* Biochemically characterize the antigen.

and cause infiltration of neutrophils from the blood. IgG1, IgG3, and IgG4 are particularly good at binding to receptors on neutrophils and macrophages through their heavy chain, thereby arming the phagocyte with a molecule on its surface that can bind bacteria. The bacteria are then "gobbled up" by the phagocyte in a process called **opsonization**. Macrophages armed with IgG antibodies can also kill target cells expressing the antigen on its surface, by **antibody-dependent cellular cytotoxicity**.

IgG antibodies are also specifically transported across the placenta to give passive immunity to neonates.

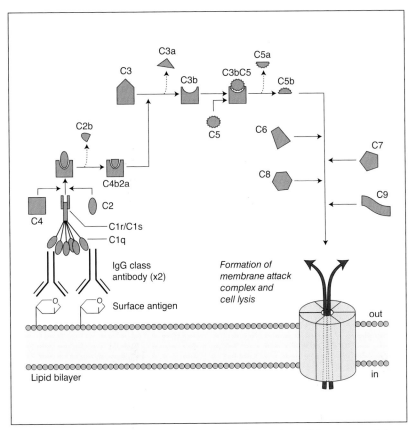

Figure 16. Antibodies bind to antigens on the cell surface and recruit the serum protein C1q. This then cleaves C4 and C2 to form a complex that activates C3 and cleaves it into C3a and C3b. C3b then cleaves C5, which then recruits other complement components to form the membrane attack complex, which punches a hole in the cell. If the hole is punched in a bacterium, the contents of the bacterial cytosol leak out through the hole and the bacterium is killed. In the example shown here, the antibody is against a mammalian cell (eg, red blood cell), but the process is similar. Ig: immunoglobulin.

IgE

Binds to receptors on mast cells and, when cross-linked by antigen, causes the mast cell to degranulate and release molecules such as histamine and 5-hydroxytryptamine, which cause the itching and reddening of allergies.

IgA

On the other hand, does not fix complement. It is the main antibody in the gut wall. It is secreted across the epithelium, where it binds to and agglutinates bacteria and viruses (**Table 1**).

	IgM	IgG	IgE	IgA
Serum concentration (mg/mL)	1.5	10	0.01	2
Fixes complement	+++++	++	–	–
Crosses placenta	–	++	–	–
Binds to mast cells	–	–	+++	–
Secretory antibody	+	–	–	+++

Table 1. The function of different antibody classes. Ig: immunoglobulin.

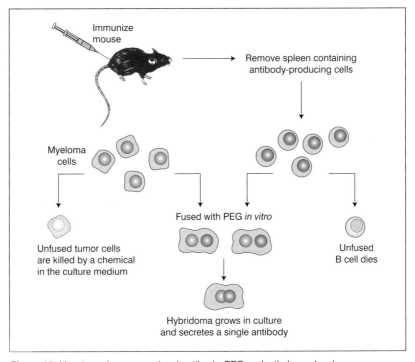

Figure 17. How to make a monoclonal antibody. PEG: polyethylene glycol.

A Beginner's Guide to Immunology

Monoclonal antibodies

In 1975, Georges JF Köhler and César Milstein discovered a way of immortalizing antibody-producing cells of single-specificity (monoclonal antibodies), for which they received the 1984 Nobel Prize. This technique revolutionized medicine. Monoclonal antibodies are now used in cancer diagnosis and therapy, immunohistochemistry, immunoassays, immunotherapy for chronic inflammation, and a host of other applications. The techniques involved in making a monoclonal antibody are shown in **Figure 17**.

So many antibodies were made, which identified so many structures, that a system of nomenclature was devised to avoid confusion. **Box 4** discusses the CD system of classifying antibodies and molecules.

2 A Beginner's Guide to Gut Immunology

Introduction

The gut presents a particular problem to the immune system. To be able to absorb food, the gut needs to have a thin epithelial lining. The small intestine has a huge number of finger-like villi, which gives the epithelial lining an area of over 400 m^2. It is made up of absorptive epithelial cells and mucus-secreting goblet cells, a few endocrine cells and Paneth cells. The linings of the stomach and colon are also only one cell thick, whereas the esophagus has a squamous multilayered epithelium (**Figure 1**).

Despite the presence of stomach acid, which kills most bacteria and viruses, many infectious diseases use the oral route to colonize the gut or to reach the thin epithelium, which is an easily breached portal of entry into the body. At the same time, we also eat large amounts of food proteins, and our ileum and colon contain 100,000 billion microbes with which we live in harmony. The principal problem for the gut immune system, therefore, is how to recognize pathogens in the face of noise from food and the normal bacterial flora, and how to prevent immune responses to food and the normal flora. This is a delicate balance, and failure to achieve it results in disease.

Because of these factors, the gut has a very active immune system that is fundamentally different from the systemic immune system.

Organized lymphoid structures of the gut

Antigens from food and bacteria can cross the healthy gut epithelium and enter the blood in amounts sufficient to elicit an antibody response. In itself, this is insufficient to produce disease – for example, all bottle-fed babies have very high

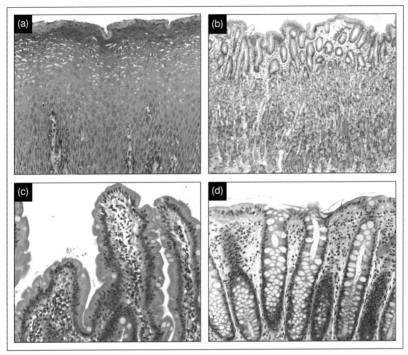

Figure 1. Histology of the different parts of the bowel. (**a**) The typical appearance of the esophagus, which has a squamous epithelium, many cells thick. In contrast, the stomach (**b**) is lined by just a single layer of epithelial cells. The surface area of the small bowel (**c**) is huge because of the millions of finger-like villi, also lined by a single layer of epithelium. Finally, the colon (**d**) has a thin mucosa lined by a single epithelial layer that contains many mucus-secreting goblet cells.

Hematoxylin and eosin stains. (**a**) Magnification ×200. (**b–d**) Magnification ×200.

levels of IgG antibodies to cow's milk proteins and yet suffer no adverse effects. Antigens cross in two places:

- across the columnar epithelium of the villus, where they enter the lamina propria (LP) and then diffuse into the blood
- into the lymphoid tissues

There is more lymphoid tissue in the gut than in the rest of the body combined. The organized lymphoid tissue of the small intestine was first described by Johann Conrad Peyer in 1677. The lymphoid structures of the gastrointestinal tract have anatomic features in common that distinguish them from other secondary lymphoid tissues. The most obvious of these common features is the lack of a defined capsule or afferent lymphatics.

A Beginner's Guide to Gut Immunology

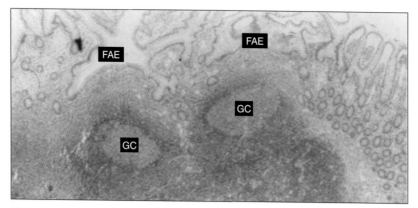

Figure 2. Histologic section of a Peyer's patch from a healthy individual. Note the large GCs, where B cells are responding to luminal antigens. In addition, the FAE overlying the dome is clearly visible. FAE: follicle-associated epithelium; GC: germinal center. Hematoxylin and eosin stain. Magnification ×40.

Peyer's patches

The best characterized of the lymphoid tissues are the PPs of the terminal ileum (**Figure 2**), but similar structures exist in the colon as isolated follicles. Structurally, PPs are organized areas of lymphoid tissue in the mucosa of the small bowel. They are overlain by a specialized lymphoepithelium (the follicle-associated epithelium [FAE]) that lacks both crypts and villi. By late adolescence there are about 225–300 PPs in the whole small intestine, although this number decreases with increasing age.

The FAE is derived from crypts of Lieberkuhn adjacent to the follicles. FAE is different from columnar villus epithelium in that it is cuboidal and contains few goblet cells. In addition, FAE contains specialized microfold or 'M' cells, also derived from adjacent crypts, which have microfolds rather than microvilli on their surface (**Figure 3**). M cells have attenuated processes to adjacent cells and are very closely associated with lymphocytes (clusters of T cells and B cells lie next to M cells in the epithelium). M cells play a role in antigen entry into the dome area of the follicle (**Figure 4**). This has been clearly shown for reovirus in mice (which only adheres to and penetrates the M cells of the FAE), poliovirus, and many other antigens. Pathogenic intestinal microbes such as virulent *Salmonella* species, *Yersinia enterocolitica*, *Y. pseudotuberculosis*, and *Shigella* all take advantage of the phagocytic capacity of M cells to invade the gut mucosa.

The most prominent features of a PP are the large GCs, which are full of proliferating B cells, even in healthy individuals. These B cells respond to antigens of the normal flora and food and undergo class-switching to IgA.

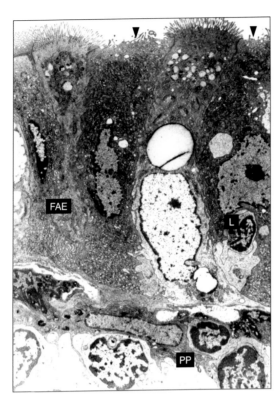

Figure 3. Electron micrograph of an M cell in the FAE overlying a human PP. There are two M cells in the image (arrowheads), both clearly identifiable because of the absence of microvilli. Note also their close association with L. FAE: follicle-associated epithelium; L: lymphocytes; PP: Peyer's patch.

Magnification ×1,000.

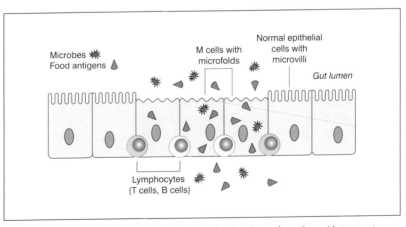

Figure 4. The function of M cells. Microbes and food antigens from the gut lumen are phagocytosed and pinocytosed by M cells in the Peyer's patch dome epithelium and transported across the epithelial barrier.

A Beginner's Guide to Gut Immunology

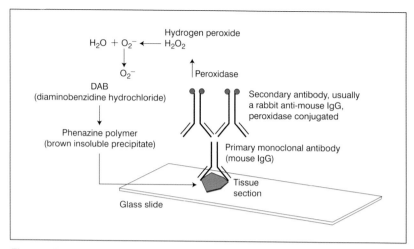

Figure 5. Immunoperoxidase histochemistry (not to scale). In immunohistochemistry, sections of tissue are placed on glass slides. They are then covered with an antibody, usually a mouse monoclonal IgG, against a structure on the surface of an immune cell. If the particular cell type is present, the antibody will bind to its antigen. The slide is then washed and incubated with another antibody (eg, a rabbit anti-mouse IgG), which has been labeled with the peroxidase enzyme. If the first antibody is in the tissue, the second antibody will bind. The slides are then washed again and hydrogen peroxide and a soluble substrate are added to the slide. Peroxidase splits H_2O_2 into water and O_2^-. The oxygen molecule reacts with the substrate and makes it insoluble, so it precipitates around the reaction – usually forming a brown color. The section is then washed and counterstained with a blue dye to visualize all the cells. Positive cells appear brown. Ig: immunoglobulin.

Immunohistochemistry (a technique to visualize molecules on the surface of cells in a tissue section using specific antibodies) allows detailed analysis of the types of cells infiltrating healthy and diseased gut. The principle of immunohistochemistry is shown in **Figure 5**. In PPs, the highest density of T cells is found in the areas surrounding the HEV between the follicles. The majority of these T cells are CD4+ (**Figure 6**).

Numerous APCs (macrophages and dendritic cells) are present in the dome area of human PPs and in the T-cell zones. The presence of dendritic cells in the dome, immediately underlying the M cells, which are MHC class II negative, suggests that, in PPs, most antigen presentation takes place in the dome region.

A striking feature of PPs is that when T cells and B cells are activated at this site, they leave after a few days and migrate via the mesenteric nodes to the blood.

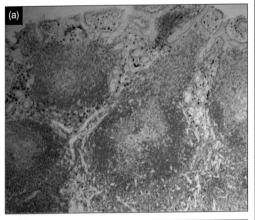

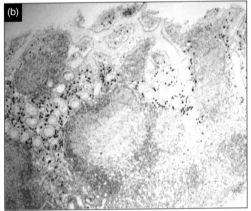

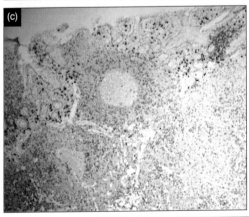

Figure 6. Immunohistologic image of a human PP stained with antibodies to (**a**) CD3 (all T cells), (**b**) CD4 (helper T cells), and (**c**) CD8 (cytotoxic T cells). CD4 cells are abundant in the areas between the B-cell follicles and also extend into the dome region. The majority of these T cells are in transit from the blood through the PP. They exit the PP through efferent lymphatics and enter the mesenteric lymph nodes. After migrating through the mesenteric nodes, they again migrate via efferent lymph into the thoracic duct and drain into the inferior vena cava.
PP: Peyer's patch.

Magnification ×100.

A Beginner's Guide to Gut Immunology

The lamina propria and the epithelium: the effector component of the mucosal immune response

A common mucosal immune system?

In the 1970s and 1980s, the notion of a common mucosal immune system was popular. The basic idea was very simple: T and B cells migrating from PPs could home to other mucosal sites, such as the breasts or lungs, and mediate immunity. Thus, oral vaccination could protect against diseases of the respiratory tree. This idea has been somewhat revised and, although there is some cross-traffic, it is now clear that the immune system of the airways and gut are somewhat different and that even the upper gut is somewhat separate from the lower gut and colon.

It has long been established that PPs are on the major route of lymphocyte recirculation. Small, virgin T cells, probably recent thymic emigrants, can enter PPs from the blood through the HEVs. Virgin B cells are also present in the area surrounding the follicle and in the dome region. When these T and B cells become activated in PPs by gut antigens, they differentiate locally for a few days, and then leave the PPs via the afferent lymphatics as large T- and B-cell blasts.

These cells enter the blood via the mesenteric node and thoracic duct, and home back to the LP (**Figure 7**). This is achieved through the surface integrin α4β7. In PPs, activated T and B cells acquire α4β7. The ligand for α4β7 is mucosal addressin cell adhesion molecule (MAdCAM)1, which is present on the endothelium of blood vessels in the LP. If a cell in the blood expresses α4β7, it can bind to MAdCAM1 on the LP vessel, adhere to the surface, and squeeze through into the LP.

B cells

Once in the LP, B cells undergo terminal differentiation to become IgA plasma cells. In healthy individuals, the gut is full of IgA plasma cells (**Figure 8**). In order for IgA to reach the gut lumen, it has to be transported across the epithelium. It is estimated that 5 g of IgA is transported across the gut epithelium every day. The transport mechanism is now well worked out (**Figure 9**).

The basolateral surface of epithelial cells contains a receptor that binds J chain, the molecule that links IgA into dimers and IgM into pentamers. Accordingly, the receptor is called the polymeric Ig receptor. After binding, IgA is transcytosed across the cell and secreted into the gut lumen. IgA is cleaved from its receptor on

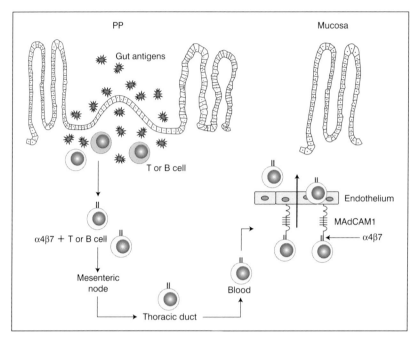

Figure 7. The migration pathway of T and B cells from the PPs of the gut to the LP. If T or B cells in a PP react with antigens from the gut lumen then they become activated, begin to express the α4β7 integrin, leave the PP, and enter the blood via the mesenteric nodes and thoracic duct. Once in the blood, they home back to the mucosa. This occurs because α4β7 integrin is the specific receptor for MAdCAM1, which is expressed in endothelial cells in the vessels of the LP. LP: lamina propria; MAdCAM1: mucosal addressin cell adhesion molecule 1; PP: Peyer's patch.

the epithelial cell, although some of the receptor remains bound to J chain (this part of the receptor is termed secretory component). IgA plasma cells in the gut only live for less than a week and are replaced by fresh cells from PPs.

T cells

In healthy individuals, the small bowel is full of T cells. T cells are also present in healthy colon, but not at the same density as in the small bowel. CD4 cells predominate in the LP and CD8 cells in the epithelium (**Figure 10**).

Lamina propria lymphocytes

CD4 T cells are also derived from PPs and use MAdCAM1 to enter the LP, and, like B cells, die within a week. CD4 T cells rarely enter the epithelium. Recent studies indicate that, in humans, LP CD4 T cells from healthy people make IFN-γ, showing that they are Th1 cells.

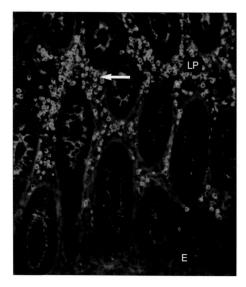

Figure 8. IgA plasma cells (**arrow**) in healthy small intestine stained green with an antibody to IgA. These are localized exclusively in the LP and never enter the epithelium. The weak staining in the epithelium of the glands is IgA being actively transported into the gut lumen. E: epithelium; Ig: immunoglobulin; LP: lamina propria.

Magnification ×100.

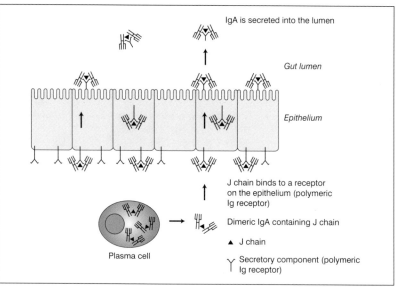

Figure 9. The mechanism by which IgA (estimated at 5 g/day) is transported across the gut epithelium. The basolateral surface of epithelial cells contains a receptor (secretory component [polymeric Ig receptor]) that binds J chain, the molecule that links IgA into dimers and IgM into pentamers. Through J chain, the IgA dimer binds to this receptor, is transcytosed across the cell, and secreted into the gut lumen. The final step involves the proteolytic cleavage of the polymeric IgA from the receptor on the apical membrane of the epithelial cell. However, a part of the receptor remains bound to J chain. When this part was discovered in the 1960s, it was called secretory component because it was found with secretory antibodies. Ig: immunoglobulin.

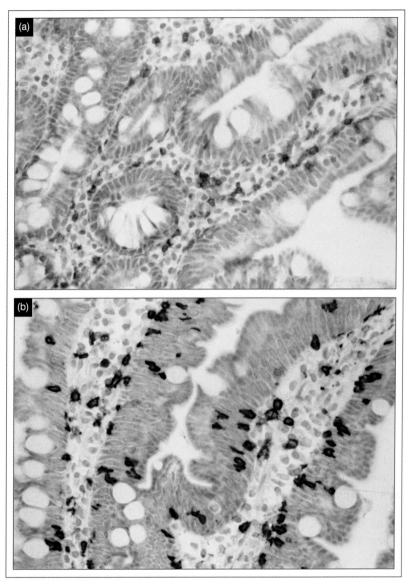

Figure 10. (a) CD4 and (b) CD8 cells in healthy small bowel. The majority of T cells in the lamina propria are CD4+. Functional studies have shown that these are activated cells that secrete interferon γ, even in healthy individuals. The majority of T cells in the epithelium are CD8+. These cells are cytotoxic effectors and contain molecules that can lyse other cells. The control of this function *in vivo* is not known. Epithelial lymphocytes are unusual in that they are long lived (persisting as the epithelium is renewed around them) and are made up of only a few T-cell clones.

Magnification ×400.

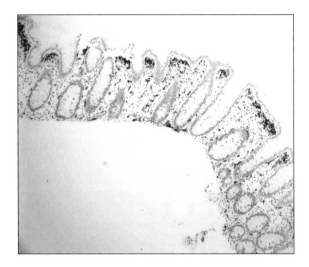

Figure 11.
Macrophages in the intestine stained with CD68 antibody. In particular, note the band of macrophages immediately below the epithelium. These are highly phagocytic cells that probably kill colonic bacteria that cross the epithelium.

Magnification ×100.

Intraepithelial lymphocytes

The lymphocytes in the gut epithelium (intraepithelial lymphocytes [IELs]) are nearly all CD8 T cells and it is not clear if they come from PPs. They are probably quite long lived, and remain in the epithelium as the enterocytes flow past them to be extruded from the villus tips. IELs are unusual in that they are the only cell type in the body that, when isolated and studied *in vitro*, can be shown to be constitutively cytotoxic. Clearly, some interaction in the epithelium prevents them from killing adjacent epithelial cells, but the mechanism of this is unknown.

IELs are also unusual in that they express a very limited number of T-cell clones. In normal T-cell populations TCR usage is random, with lots of different Vα and Vβs being used. In mouse and human IELs, however, only a few clones dominate, making up 20%–50% of the cells. These persist over time and over long stretches of bowel. IELs are also enriched for γδ T cells, even in healthy individuals, and are particularly abundant in celiac disease. A role for these cells in the gut remains to be characterized, although they might be important in killing infected epithelial cells.

Taken together – because of the large size of the gut and the huge surface area of the bowel (400 m^2) – the number of T cells in the epithelium and LP of healthy individuals exceeds that of the systemic tissues. The LP also contains large numbers of macrophages (especially in the colon, **Figure 11**), dendritic cells, and some mast cells and eosinophils.

Is the gut tolerant or unresponsive to food and normal bacteria?

There is a general misconception that the gut is an unresponsive site – ie, that because everyone does not have gut disease, we must somehow be tolerant to what we eat. This notion has arisen for a number of reasons, but mainly because of the phenomenon of oral tolerance (**Figure 12**). If you feed a mouse a foreign protein antigen and then, a few weeks later, immunize it with the same antigen systemically, the animal will not respond immunologically (especially the T-cell arm of the immune response). This is called oral tolerance, but is more correctly termed orally induced systemic unresponsiveness, since the immunization is systemic, not oral. While it may be a way of preventing systemic responses to antigens that enter the blood, there is actually no evidence that feeding antigens prevents mucosal responses in humans.

The fact that the gut is filled with T cells and B cells in healthy individuals, and that both the IgA system and the T-cell system in the LP are highly activated, suggests that there is an ongoing response to food and bacteria. It could be argued that these are responses to subclinical infections, but studies in mice have clearly shown that benign gut bacteria can elicit large mucosal immune responses. We would therefore argue that the gut does not maintain a state of tolerance to food and normal bacteria, but instead preserves a disease-free state often known as physiological inflammation.

What is the function of T and B cells in the healthy gut?

It is well established that IgA can protect the gut from infection. By binding to microbes, it can prevent them from coming into contact with epithelial cells and colonizing the surface of the gut (eg, pathogenic *Escherichia coli*) or invading the cell (eg, rotavirus). However, it is highly controversial as to whether IgA plays a role in healthy individuals in the western world. IgA deficiency is common, but does not predispose to intestinal infections because there is a compensatory enhanced mucosal IgM response. Patients with agammaglobulinemia do suffer from gut infections such as *Giardia*, but it is not known if this is due to the lack of secretory IgA and IgM or serum IgG. Likewise, all individuals make IgA to their own gut microbes and most bacteria in stools are covered in IgA, but there is little evidence that this IgA prevents the normal bacteria from invading the tissues.

A Beginner's Guide to Gut Immunology

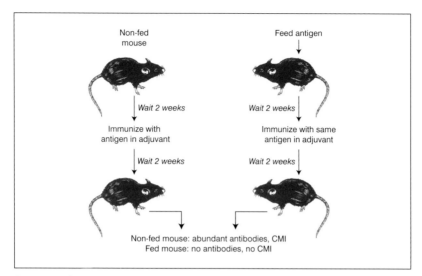

Figure 12. Oral tolerance. This is a very well characterized phenomenon in rodents, with only limited studies in humans. If you feed an antigen to a mouse or rat, and 2 weeks later try to immunize the animal with the same antigen systemically, it will only make a weak response compared with an animal that was not previously fed. Oral tolerance has been tried as a strategy to prevent food hypersensitivity and autoimmune disease in humans, but the results have been disappointing. This phenomenon is misnamed – it is more correctly termed "orally-induced systemic unresponsiveness". CMI: cell-mediated immunity.

For T cells, the situation is even more confusing. The healthy human intestine is filled with activated T cells. When these are depleted, especially CD4 cells in AIDS, patients acquire gut infections. However, the mechanisms by which CD4 cells in healthy people keep the gut free from infection are not known – animal models have clearly shown a role for CD4 cells in resistance to pathogens such as *Toxoplasma gondii*, mouse enteropathogenic *E. coli*, and *Helicobacter felis*, but the detailed mechanisms are still unclear.

3 A Beginner's Guide to Immune-mediated Inflammation

Introduction

A great challenge for the immune system is to achieve a balance between destroying infections and infected cells without damaging normal cells and tissues. In reality, tissue damage is unavoidable in the course of protective immunity – it is really the extent of the damage that is important. In the 1950s, Gell and Coombs classified tissue-damaging immune responses (ie, hypersensitivity) into four types, which still form a useful paradigm today.

Hypersensitivity

Type I

Mechanism

Type I, or immediate, hypersensitivity involves IgE. The bulk of IgE is tightly bound to the surfaces of mast cells, where it can remain for several months, with only trace amounts in serum. Antigen binding to surface IgE on mast cells cross-links the IgE molecules, and triggers degranulation of the mast cell and, within minutes, release of preformed mediators (**Figure 1**). These mediators include histamine, serotonin, proteases, and eosinophil and neutrophil chemotactic factors. They cause vascular permeability, mucus secretion, vasodilation, infiltration of inflammatory cells, edema, and smooth muscle cell contraction.

The mast cell also releases cytokines such as TNFα and IL-5 (a potent eosinophil chemoattractant and growth factor), which recruit more inflammatory cells.

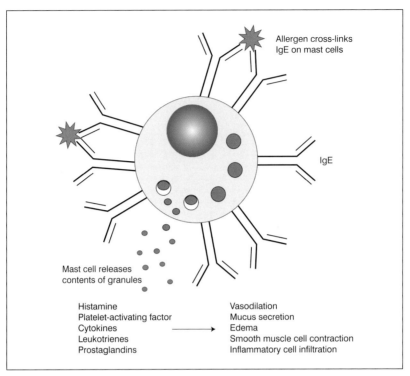

Figure 1. Type I hypersensitivity is mediated by allergens binding to IgE on mast cells. It is important that the allergen binds to several IgE molecules at the same time. Binding signals the mast cell to release preformed mediators (eg, histamine), which are contained in granules within the cell. The cell then starts to synthesize leukotrienes and prostaglandins. The net effect of these inflammatory mediators is vasodilation, mucus secretion, edema, smooth muscle cell contraction, and an influx of inflammatory cells into the tissues. Ig: immunoglobulin.

After activation, the mast cell also makes inflammatory molecules, such as leukotrienes and prostaglandins from arachidonic acid, which cause smooth muscle contraction and increasedvascular permeability.

Type I hypersensitivity is due to the overactivity of Th2 cells, which make excess IL-4 and IL-5. IL-4 is the cytokine that drives IgE production by B cells. Why some people make Th2 responses to antigens such as pollen is not known, but there is a clear genetic predisposition towards such a response.

Effect

Individuals who make this kind of response are termed atopic or allergic, and make up about 5–10% of the population. In most people, allergies are minor (eg, hay fever), but highly atopic individuals can generate such severe responses

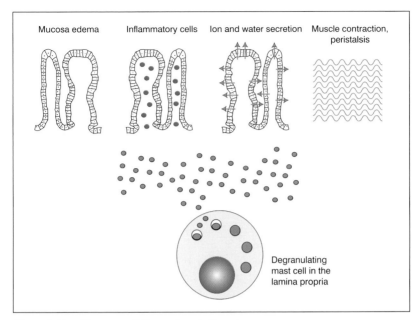

Mucosa edema   Inflammatory cells   Ion and water secretion   Muscle contraction, peristalsis

Degranulating mast cell in the lamina propria

Figure 2. Type I hypersensitivity reactions in the gut.

that they go into systemic anaphylactic shock and die. Peanut allergies are particularly dangerous.

Type I hypersensitivity reactions to food can cause problems in the gut. There is very little morphologic damage during an acute immediate hypersensitivity reaction, but mast cell products cause fluid secretion, mucus release, eosinophil infiltration, and increased peristalsis, resulting in diarrhea (**Figure 2**).

Type II

Mechanism

Type II hypersensitivity is caused by antibodies directed against cell surface antigens. The classic example is Rhesus incompatibility, which causes hemolytic disease of the newborn. Rhesus antigens are found on red blood cells. If a Rhesus-negative mother gives birth to a Rhesus-positive child (because the father is Rhesus-positive), then, at birth, some of the neonate's red blood cells enter the mother's circulation and stimulate the mother to make IgG anti-Rhesus antibodies. If the fetus in subsequent pregnancies is Rhesus-positive, IgG antibodies cross the placenta and enter the child's circulation where they bind to red blood cells, fix complement, and lyse red blood cells.

Another classic example is autoimmune hemolytic anemia, where autoantibodies against red blood cells fix complement and lyse red blood cells. This process is fast (usually 10–20 minutes).

Effect
Type II hypersensitivity reactions are not well defined in the gut. In pernicious anemia (see p. 121), autoantibodies probably kill parietal cells through a type II hypersensitivity reaction. There is also some evidence that autoantibodies to epithelial cells are important in ulcerative colitis (UC) (see p. 142).

Type III

Mechanism
Type III hypersensitivity is caused by antibody–antigen complexes. Every time an antibody meets its specific antigen in the blood or tissues it forms a complex. Usually, this complex is removed from the blood by macrophages in the liver and spleen, or engulfed by a tissue phagocyte. In certain situations, however – such as in persistent infection, autoimmune disease, and chronic exposure to the antigen (eg, inhalation) – immune complexes are deposited in blood vessel walls and tissues. Complement is activated locally, and, because C3a and C5a (breakdown components of complement activation) are highly chemotactic for neutrophils, this results in neutrophils moving into the tissues. The neutrophils degranulate and release enzymes and free radicals, which cause increased vascular permeability and cell damage.

Effect
Serum sickness is caused by immune complexes forming in the blood. It is so called because it occurs after the injection of large amounts of serum (eg, horse anti-diphtheria serum). While the sera neutralizes diphtheria toxin, the recipient makes antibodies to horse proteins, which results in immune complexes. These then deposit in the basement membranes of the joints and kidneys, fix complement, attract neutrophils, and cause disease. This is a particular problem in the kidney where immune complexes can damage the blood vessels leading to kidney failure (**Figure 3**).

Serum sickness also occurs in patients who make antibodies to the mouse components of anti-TNFα antibodies (eg, infliximab). In second and subsequent infusions, the human anti-mouse antibodies form a complex with the anti-TNFα antibodies and deposit in tissues.

The Arthus reaction occurs when immune complexes form in tissues, complement is activated, and neutrophils are drawn into the region, resulting

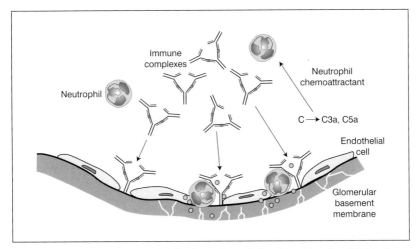

Figure 3. As immune complexes in blood pass through the glomerulus, they bind to the basement membrane between endothelial cells. They fix complement, and C3a and C5a are released. This attracts circulating neutrophils from the blood into the endothelial layer where they secrete molecules which damage the endothelium and basement membrane.

in an edematous swelling. In UC, there is some evidence that the massive neutrophil infiltration into the tissues is due to a local Arthus reaction.

In most cases, immune complex diseases are due to chronic exposure to antigen, such as anti-DNA antibodies in systemic lupus erythematosus. Other diseases that are classically associated with type III hypersensitivity include glomerulonephritis, arthritis, and farmer's lung.

Type IV

Mechanism
Type IV hypersensitivity is mediated by T cells. It is best exemplified by the induration and swelling seen in the skin of individuals infected with tuberculosis (TB) when antigens from the tubercle bacillus are injected intradermally into the skin (**Figure 4**). The swelling takes 24–48 hours to occur, and so type IV hypersensitivity is also called delayed-type hypersensitivity.

In the example shown in **Figure 4**, when antigen is injected into the skin, it is taken up by Langerhans cells (dendritic-type cells) and the peptides are presented to T cells in association with MHC class II molecules (see **Chapter 1**). In individuals with TB, memory cells sensitized to TB antigens recirculate around the body. Eventually, one will recognize the peptide on the Langerhans cell. The T cell then releases cytokines such as IFNγ, macrophage migration

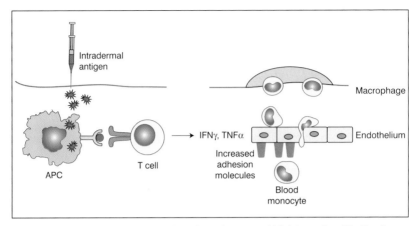

Figure 4. Type IV hypersensitivity (delayed-type hypersensitivity) is mediated by T cells. When antigen is injected into the skin, it is presented to circulating T cells by Langerhans cells in the dermis. The T cells release cytokines (eg, IFNγ and TNFα), which increase adhesion molecules on the endothelium. Circulating monocytes bind to the activated endothelium and migrate into the skin. Because type IV hypersensitivity causes a cellular infiltrate, the swelling it causes is hard and indurated. If the antigen persists and continues to drive a cell-mediated immune response, the macrophages can fuse, become epithelioid giant cells, and form granulomata. APC: antigen-presenting cell; IFN: interferon; TNF: tumor necrosis factor.

inhibitory factor, IL-2, and TNFα, which increase the expression of adhesion molecules on the surrounding vessel walls. When monocytes pass through these blood vessels, they stick to the vessel endothelium and migrate out of the blood into the tissue. Type IV hypersensitivity is mediated by Th1 cells: these have a characteristic cytokine profile, namely IFNγ and TNFα.

Effect

Type IV reactions are very destructive in humans. If the antigen persists then T cells and macrophages destroy the tissue, which is then replaced by a scar. If the antigen cannot be destroyed, the macrophages will eventually wall it off in a granuloma, which is where an organized accumulation of macrophages differentiate into epithelioid giant cells (**Figure 5**). If the bacteria continue to replicate in the granuloma, as in TB, there is a lot of cell death and the granuloma becomes filled with caseous material (the contents are semi-solid or thick and cheesy, hence *caseous* from casein, the milk protein). If the antigen does not replicate, but is hard to break down, non-caseating granulomata form.

Crohn's disease (see p. 86) is a Th1 delayed-type hypersensitivity disease associated with granuloma. Humans are especially good at making type IV reactions – much better, for example, than rodents.

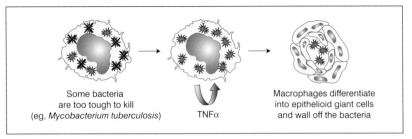

| Some bacteria are too tough to kill (eg, *Mycobacterium tuberculosis*) | TNFα | Macrophages differentiate into epithelioid giant cells and wall off the bacteria |

Figure 5. Granulomata are a feature of type IV (delayed-type) hypersensitivity reactions. They are classically associated with TB, where the immune system walls off the bacteria into caseating granulomata. Granuloma formation critically depends on an autocrine TNFα loop, which drives giant-cell formation. One of the unforeseen consequences of anti-TNFα therapy has been the deaths of patients with latent TB. When TNFα is neutralized to help treat Crohn's disease or rheumatoid arthritis, it also leads to the dissolution of granulomata. The bacteria then escape and multiply unchecked in the host. TB: tuberculosis; TNF: tumor necrosis factor.

The immunological basis for tissue inflammation

In healthy individuals, most tissues of the body contain few inflammatory cells. An exception is the gut, and to some extent the lungs, where inflammatory cells are present even in health. In order to get into the tissues, macrophages, lymphocytes, and neutrophils have to move out of the blood vessels and into the tissues: a process called extravasation. It needs to be remembered that this mechanism evolved to deal with infections in tissues, and so there is a need to be able to mobilize large numbers of phagocytic cells into the tissues where they can engulf and kill invading bacteria.

Mechanism
When bacteria invade the tissues they are recognized by serum-derived molecules such as mannose-binding lectin which can activate and complement itself, and by TLRs on resident cells. Activation through these receptors causes the resident cells to secrete cytokines such as IL-1β and TNFα. These cytokines then act in the local environment to increase the expression of adhesion molecules on the endothelial cells of blood vessels (**Figure 6**). Products of the complement cascade also mobilize cells into tissue.

Adhesion molecules include P-selectin, E-selectin, and ICAM-1. Monocytes (blood macrophages), lymphocytes, and neutrophils have cell-surface receptors for these vascular adhesion molecules. As they pass through the blood vessel they can therefore bind to the vessel wall and migrate into the tissues.

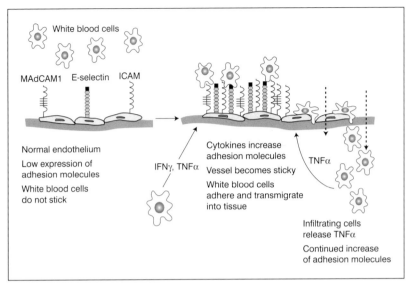

Figure 6. Endothelial adhesion molecules control the migration of cells from the blood into tissues during chronic inflammation. In the example shown, a blood vessel in the gut expresses low amounts of adhesion molecules (MAdCAM1, E-selectin, and ICAM). Consequently, white cells in the blood (which have receptors for these molecules) pass through the tissues. When activated by IFNγ or TNFα from T cells, the blood vessel increases the amount of adhesion molecules it expresses on its surface. With more adhesion molecules, there is a greater chance they will bind to receptors on the white cell surface and deliver a signal telling the cell to squeeze through the vessel wall and into the tissue. Once in the tissue, the infiltrating cells will secrete TNFα and continue the cycle. ICAM: intercellular cell adhesion molecule; IFN: interferon; MAdCAM1: mucosal addressin cell adhesion molecule 1; TNF: tumor necrosis factor.

The infiltrate is classified as acute if it is full of neutrophils because these are short-lived in tissues (hours to a few days) and chronic if it is full of monocyte-derived macrophages and lymphocytes, which live for days or weeks.

Inflammation can be both local and systemic. Thus, when you get an infection, cells at the site of infection release, among others, IL-1β, IL-6, and TNFα:

- IL-1β can pass into the blood and act on receptors in the brain to make you feel hot and give you a fever.
- IL-6 binds to hepatocytes and induces them to make C-reactive protein (CRP). CRP is a useful marker of inflammation and has many functions. It can activate complement, bind to bacterial cell walls, and increase phagocytosis.
- TNFα also works on the brain to suppress appetite, and induces cachexia (where the body breaks down proteins rather than synthesizes them).

A Beginner's Guide to Immune-mediated Inflammation

At the local level in the inflamed site, TNFα and IL-1β also act on the blood vessels to increase the number of adhesion molecules and bring even more inflammatory cells into the site to combat the infection. IL-1β (which is made by macrophages) also has an important function in primary T-cell responses.

Effect

Ideally, phagocytes, together with antibodies and T cells, will eliminate the infection. With the stimulus gone, the inflammatory cells will eventually die and the tissue returns to normal. If, however, the infection is not resolved, then more and more inflammatory cells move into the tissue. There, they release so many toxic molecules that they can destroy the tissue itself. In particular, if T cells become chronically activated by persistent antigens then they continue to secrete TNFα and IFNγ, which then continue to increase adhesion molecules on endothelial cells and draw inflammatory cells into the tissues. This is a particular problem in autoimmune disease, where the antigen is a self antigen and so cannot be destroyed without removing its function, such as myelin basic protein in the brain or collagen in the joint.

In Crohn's disease, where it is thought that the immune response is directed against the bacterial flora, the persistence of the flora leads to the persistence of the inflammation. One way to stop tissue damage in diseases such as Crohn's disease or rheumatoid arthritis would therefore be to block the expression of adhesion molecules on blood vessels so that blood-borne inflammatory cells remain in the circulation. This can be done with specific antibodies against vascular adhesion molecules and has been successful in patients with Crohn's disease.

Chemokines

The most recently discovered family of molecules is the chemokines. These are small molecular-weight polypeptides that bind to specific receptors on different cell types and exert their biological effects. So far, over 20 chemokine receptors and over 40 chemokines have been described. As their name implies, they cause inflammatory cells to undergo chemotaxis, ie, move along a gradient of molecules in a directional fashion. Examples:

- IL-8, one of the first chemokines discovered, is highly chemotactic for neutrophils and draws them into tissues.
- Eotaxin, which is made by a variety of cell types, attracts eosinophils into tissues and, not surprisingly, is highly expressed in allergic individuals.

The function of chemokines and their receptors, however, goes beyond inflammation. They can also function as surface receptors for viruses, eg, for HIV. They are important in the migration of cells around the body and are also involved in angiogenesis (the growth of new blood vessels).

Negative effects

A final and unwanted consequence of inflammation in tissues is that it predisposes to malignancy. Free radicals can directly damage DNA. Increased cell proliferation, for example of epithelial cells in the gut wall as a consequence of inflammatory bowel disease (IBD), will increase the possibility of a random mutation occurring in epithelial cells as the cells replicate their DNA.

A-Z Disease Listing

Allergic proctocolitis (usually due to cows' milk)

Cause	An IgE-mediated allergic reaction to food, including cows' milk proteins and soy proteins.
Age of onset	Most common in children. It can even be seen in exclusively breast-fed neonates who become sensitized to the dietary cows' milk in their mother's milk.
Principal clinical features	Vomiting, diarrhea, abdominal pain, rectal bleeding, and anemia.
Epidemiology/genetics	Relatively uncommon. No known genetic basis, other than the genetic tendency to develop allergies.
Association with other diseases	There may be associated atopy in other tissues (eg, asthma, eczema).
Location of lesion within bowel	Any part of the large intestine, but the sigmoid colon and rectum are most commonly involved (**Figure 1**).
Extraintestinal manifestations	None, other than those associated with atopy.
Diagnostic tests	Definitive diagnosis can only be achieved through an elimination diet and challenge, but this is very rarely carried out since most infants thrive on a milk-free diet.
Major immunopathologic features	Colonoscopy reveals mucosal erythema and, in severe cases, ulceration. Colonic biopsy classically reveals intense eosinophilic infiltration of the LP and muscularis mucosa. Peripheral eosinophilia is also commonly present. Features of chronicity (as seen in IBD) such as glandular distortion are not seen. Serum IgE levels are often raised.
Putative immunopathogenesis	It is not clear why allergic proctocolitis manifests in the colon in some infants, especially when considering breast-fed neonates. These infants receive minute amounts of allergen by mouth, which is unlikely to reach the distal bowel and

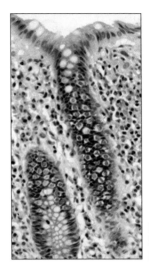

Figure 1. In allergic proctocolitis, there is marked infiltration of the lamina propria with eosinophils. Hematoxylin and eosin stain. Magnification ×400.

induce a local response. As in all food allergies, the immaturity of the intestinal mucosal barrier might allow excess amounts of allergen to enter the circulation to produce an IgE response, but there must be a major host genetic response since all infants show some deficit in barrier function and antigen penetrates into the blood in quite large amounts in all bottle-fed neonates.

It is now clear that children are born with a T-h2-type cytokine response, which switches to a Th1 response after birth. Thus, infants may produce a lot of IL-4, which will make B cells responding to antigens switch to making IgE rather than IgG. A delay in this switch might predispose some infants to this condition. Very low doses of antigen might also predispose towards an IgE-producing Th2 response.

Treatment

Changing to a hypoallergenic milk formula is often effective and usually produces a good clinical response. For infants who are sensitized through breast milk, the mother can commence a milk-free diet.

Amyloidosis

Cause	Deposition of fibrillar proteinaceous material within tissues.
Age of onset	Amyloid deposition is most common in late middle-aged and elderly patients.
Principal clinical features	These depend upon the distribution and extent of amyloid deposition, as well as the presence of underlying disease. Amyloidosis within the gut can be asymptomatic or minimally symptomatic until late in the disease process. More advanced disease might present as malabsorption, diarrhea, abdominal pain, weight loss, protein-losing enteropathy, or gut motility disorders. "Tumoral" amyloid can cause bowel obstruction.
Epidemiology/genetics	Unknown
Association with other diseases	Amyloidosis most commonly occurs in association with low-grade B-cell neoplasms, eg, lymphoma (amyloid light chain amyloid, where the amyloid deposition is made up of Ig light chains), or with chronic systemic inflammatory diseases, eg, IBD, TB, and rheumatoid arthritis (amyloid-associated protein [AA] amyloid, where the amyloid deposition is made up of acute-phase reactant products, such as serum amyloid A). Other associations include hemodialysis (β2 microglobulin). Amyloidosis can also occur as a familial condition (eg, transthyretin in familial Mediterranean fever) or as an age-related phenomenon (eg, senile cardiac amyloidosis). Since one of the precursors for tissue amyloid is serum amyloid A, an acute-phase protein made by the liver, there is an association with chronic inflammation.
Location of lesion within bowel	Any part of the gut. Deposition most commonly begins within the blood vessel walls and beneath the surface epithelium, but advanced cases can show extensive deposition within the LP and muscularis mucosa (**Figure 2**).

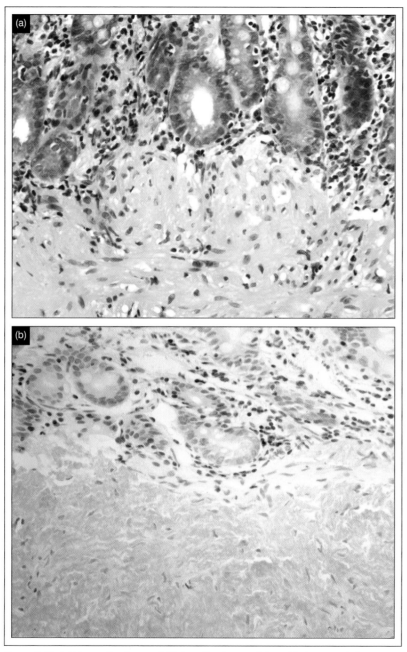

Figure 2. Rectal biopsy showing amyloid deposition in association with the muscularis mucosa. (**a**) Hematoxylin and eosin stain. Magnification ×400. (**b**) Congo red stain. Magnification ×400.

Extraintestinal manifestations	Amyloidosis can be localized or widespread, with the most common sites for the latter including the heart, lungs, and lymphoreticular system.
Diagnostic tests	Elevated serum amyloid A, a precursor of the amyloid protein in tissues, is diagnostic and can be detected with a simple laboratory test. Advanced disease may be revealed as mucosal/bowel wall thickening on radiologic and endoscopic examination. Histologic diagnosis relies upon the identification of amyloid protein within biopsy specimens.
Major immunopathologic features	Rectal biopsies are commonly taken to search for evidence of amyloidosis. Special histochemical stains such as Congo red and immunohistochemical stains such as those for AA, Ig light chains, and P component can help to confirm the presence of amyloid and determine its type. In this situation, it is important to include submucosal tissue (ie, submucosal blood vessels) if evidence of early disease is to be found.
Putative immunopathogenesis	It is not known why some people develop amyloidosis. Amyloid is a protein with a β-pleated sheet secondary structure, in which the individual subunits may comprise one of several proteins that are present in excess quantities.
	Amyloid protein can be distributed extracellularly in a localized or widespread manner, and almost any organ can be affected. Early amyloid deposition commonly occurs within blood vessel walls and nerves, while massive deposits might lead to enlargement of the affected organ with severe functional impairment or "amyloid tumor" formation. The pathological sequelae of amyloid deposition depend on the severity and distribution of the deposition – eg, cardiac amyloidosis can lead to cardiomyopathy and cardiac failure, renal amyloidosis to nephrotic syndrome, and intestinal involvement to a spectrum of clinical sequelae, including malabsorption (see above). The prognosis of widespread advanced amyloidosis is generally

poor, even if the underlying disease process is identified and treated.

| Treatment | Amyloid deposition is irreversible, but a careful search for potentially treatable underlying disease (see above) is essential. |

Autoimmune enteropathy

Cause	Unknown
Age of onset	Infancy, and occasionally in older children.
Principal clinical features	Intractable diarrhea unresponsive to dietary management.
Epidemiology/genetics	Rare. Often occurs in children of related parents.
Association with other diseases	Other autoimmune diseases, such as pernicious anemia, insulin-dependent diabetes mellitus, autoimmune hepatitis, and autoimmune thyroid disease.
Location of lesion within bowel	Small bowel or colon (**Figure 3**).
Extraintestinal manifestations	None directly, but it is associated with other autoimmune diseases.
Diagnostic tests	Approximately 50% of patients possess circulating anti-epithelial cell antibodies.
Major immunopathologic features	The small-bowel lesion bears close similarities to celiac disease. Small-bowel biopsy reveals villous atrophy, crypt hyperplasia, and increased numbers of chronic inflammatory cells within the LP and epithelium. IEL numbers are not raised and $\gamma\delta$ T cell levels are not increased. Colonic biopsy reveals mucosal glandular atrophy and increased numbers of chronic inflammatory cells within the LP. However, these changes can be subtle and patchy in nature.

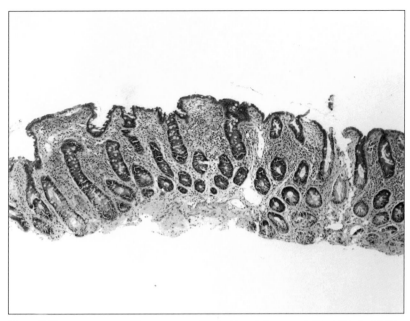

Figure 3. The appearance of the upper small bowel in autoimmune enteropathy is similar to celiac disease. However, intraepithelial lymphocyte levels are not increased. Hematoxylin and eosin stain. Magnification ×100.

Putative immunopathogenesis

Although patients often have antiepithelial cell antibodies, these do not appear to be pathogenic since they are only seen in 50% of cases. Instead, it is more probable that the disease is due to an LP CD4 Th1 response to some unidentified (perhaps self) antigen. The LP contains large numbers of activated T cells and the epithelium is strongly HLA class II positive. The rarity of this condition has so far precluded detailed immunologic investigation.

Treatment

The disease is often refractory to treatment, progressive, and usually fatal. Immunosuppressive therapy is the main treatment, eg, cyclosporin A, steroids, or azathioprine. Replacement vitamin B_{12} therapy might be required if there is coexistent pernicious anemia.

Behçet's disease

Cause	Unknown
Age of onset	Often in the second and third decades of life.
Gender bias	The male to female ratio is 2:1.
Principal clinical features	Classically associated with genital and oral ulceration, often with eye lesions. Colitis is the most common presentation within the gastrointestinal tract. Severe disease can be associated with widespread and intractable intestinal ulceration.
Epidemiology/genetics	More common in Japan than other countries. There is an association with HLA-B51.
Association with other diseases	None
Location of lesion within bowel	The disease can affect the small intestine and colon, with the most common pattern being involvement of the terminal ileum and cecum.
Extraintestinal manifestations	Many organ systems can be involved, but the most common additional conditions are arthritis, oro-genital ulceration, and iritis.
Diagnostic tests	For Behçet's disease in general, the international criteria for diagnosis require the presence of recurrent oral ulcers and two of the following:

* recurrent genital ulcers
* skin lesions
* eye lesions
* positive pathergy test (a vesicular lesion that occurs within 1–2 days of pricking the skin with a needle)

Confident diagnosis may be difficult and is largely based on the clinical pattern of organ involvement.

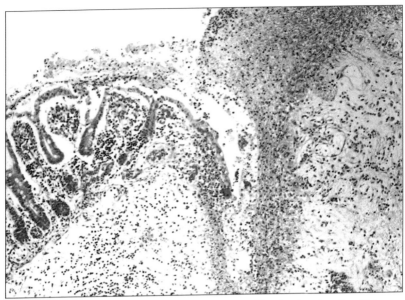

Figure 4. Small bowel showing active Behçet's disease with extensive ulceration. The characteristic lymphocytic vasculitis is often difficult to identify and, indeed, cannot be seen clearly in this illustration.
Hematoxylin and eosin stain. Magnification ×200.

Major immunopathologic features

The underlying pathology is vasculitis involving the small and large blood vessels. Biopsy might reveal mucosal ulceration associated with lymphocytic vasculitis, although the latter is not always seen and is in itself a non-specific finding (**Figure 4**).

Putative immunopathogenesis

It is unclear whether Behçet's disease is an autoimmune disease or whether it is triggered by microbial infection. Lesions in the gut can be seen as the gastrointestinal manifestations of a generalized inflammatory response at various sites throughout the body.

Treatment

Medical therapies include steroids, colchicine, cyclosporin A, thalidomide, and chlorambucil. Infliximab, an anti-TNF-α drug, has also been shown to be efficacious in severe disease.

Campylobacter enterocolitis

Cause	*Campylobacter* infection of the intestine. These Gram-negative spiral bacteria may be food- or water-borne. Three main species are pathogenic in humans: *C. jejuni, C. coli,* and *C. fetus.*
Age of onset	Any, but typically children and young adults – the ages at which Crohn's disease is also at peak incidence (see p. 86).
Principal clinical features	The incubation period is 2–5 days. Infection can be asymptomatic, but the main features of symptomatic disease are acute onset of bloody diarrhea together with abdominal pain and fever. *C. fetus* causes a more serious systemic infection that can be fatal.
Epidemiology/genetics	Campylobacters are some of the most commonly isolated stool pathogens. Outbreaks can occur in association with contaminated water supplies. Food (especially organic chickens) is also an important source of transmission. *C. jejuni* is a common cause of "traveler's diarrhea".
Association with other diseases	There is some recent evidence that *Campylobacter* infection can lead to the development of irritable bowel syndrome in some patients.
Location of lesion within bowel	Infection primarily affects the small bowel (ie, an acute enteritis, which is the most common presentation) or the colon (ie, an acute colitis).
Extraintestinal manifestations	Guillain–Barré syndrome (an acute inflammatory demyelinating neuropathy) is an unusual but important association, which occurs due to cross-reactivity between *C. jejuni* and neural antigens. Affected patients have antimyelin antibodies.
Diagnostic tests	Definitive diagnosis is by isolation and identification of the organism in stools.
Major immunopathologic features	A diffuse enterocolitis is present. Mucosal biopsies reveal edema together with acute and chronic inflammation (**Figure 5**); granulomas may be

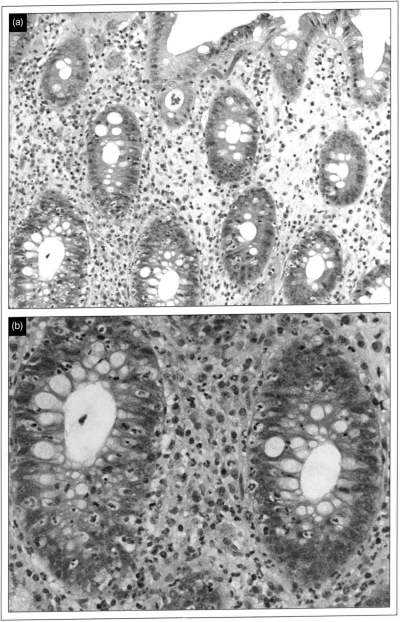

Figure 5. Rectal biopsy in *Campylobacter* infection showing an acute colitis with edema and superficial acute inflammation, but a well-preserved glandular architecture.

Hematoxylin and eosin stains. (**a**) Magnification ×200. (**b**) Magnification ×400.

present, causing potential confusion with Crohn's disease. Confirmation of the diagnosis is reliant on culture of *Campylobacter* from a stool sample.

Putative immunopathogenesis

The inflammation is directly due to invasion into the mucosa and the subsequent multiplication of *Campylobacter* organisms. The host antibacterial response results in the emigration of inflammatory cells into diseased tissue to combat the infection, with resultant collateral damage to the mucosa.

Treatment

Treatment comprises antibiotics (ciprofloxacin or erythromycin) if the patient is systemically unwell, together with supportive therapy, eg, rehydration and correction of electrolyte imbalances. Antiemetic and antidiarrheal therapy can also be used if symptoms are severe.

Carcinomas of the luminal gastrointestinal tract

Carcinomas of the luminal gastrointestinal tract most commonly arise within the esophagus, stomach, and colorectum (**Figure 6**).

Cause

Esophageal carcinoma
Invasive squamous cell carcinoma is associated with cigarette smoking, while adenocarcinoma of the lower esophagus is strongly linked to the presence of Barrett's esophagus (glandular mucosa within the lower esophagus).

Gastric carcinoma
Adenocarcinoma is associated with cigarette smoking, and the atrophic gastritis resulting from either *Helicobacter pylori* infection or pernicious anemia. There is also an increased risk of adenocarcinoma development within the gastric remnant following partial gastrectomy.

Colorectal carcinoma
Adenocarcinomas are believed to develop from dysplastic adenomas. A small percentage of

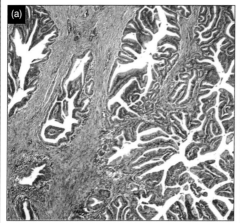

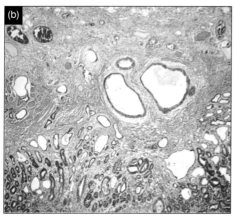

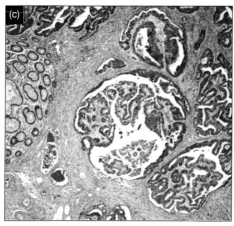

Figure 6.
(**a**) Esophageal carcinoma. Invasive adenocarcinoma of the lumenal gastrointestinal tract. Malignant glands are seen to infiltrate the muscularis propria. (**b**) Gastric carcinoma. Malignant glands are seen to infiltrate the muscularis mucosa and enter the superficial submucosa. (**c**) Colonic carcinoma. Malignant glands are seen to infiltrate the submucosa. A small quantity of normal large bowel mucosa is also present at the left edge of the photograph.

(**a–c**) Hematoxylin and eosin stains. Magnification ×40.

colorectal adenocarcinomas develop within the setting of inherited conditions, such as familial adenomatous polyposis (FAP) and hereditary nonpolyposis colorectal cancer (HNPCC).

Age of onset

Carcinomas most commonly develop during the sixth to eighth decades. Colorectal carcinomas occurring in association with FAP or HNPCC can arise in patients <50 years of age.

Principal clinical features

Carcinomas most commonly present with symptoms due to the primary tumor (eg, luminal obstruction, hemorrhage), but may also present with metastases (eg, jaundice due to liver metastases, cerebral irritation due to brain metastases) or with the general features of malignancy (eg, anorexia, general malaise).

Epidemiology/genetics

Esophageal carcinoma

Within western populations, the incidence of squamous cell carcinoma of the esophagus is reducing, while adenocarcinoma of the lower esophagus and gastro-esophageal junction is becoming more common. The increased incidence of adenocarcinoma is related to Barrett's esophagus, which is the major risk factor for this tumor. Diagnosis and treatment of gastroesophageal reflux disease might reduce the risk of carcinoma development.

Gastric and colorectal carcinoma

More common within westernized communities, with gastric carcinoma particularly common in Japan. Around 25% of colorectal carcinomas show "familial clustering", with no single identifiable inherited genetic defect. Less than 5% of colorectal cancers occur due to inherited "single-gene defects" such as FAP (due to a mutation within the adenomatous polyposis coli gene) and HNPCC (due to a mutation within one of the DNA mismatch repair enzymes, eg, hMLH-1 or hMSH-2). The development of colorectal carcinoma is associated with a stepwise accumulation of genetic defects by the colorectal epithelium, eg, mutations within the *APC, DCC* (deleted in colorectal carcinoma), k-*ras*, and *p53* genes (the "adenoma-carcinoma sequence" – see below).

Association with other diseases

Colorectal carcinoma occurring in the setting of FAP might also be associated with abdominal desmoid tumors (Gardener's syndrome) or cerebral gliomas (Turcot's syndrome). Colorectal carcinoma occurring in HNPCC can be associated with extracolonic neoplasms, such as endometrial adenocarcinoma, occurring within the same patient or a family member. There is an increased risk of colorectal carcinoma in chronic IBD, especially UC (see p. 142). Colorectal carcinoma develops from sporadic adenomas or from dysplasia-associated lesions or masses in the setting of UC (the "adenoma-carcinoma sequence"). There is growing evidence that colorectal carcinoma might develop more quickly from certain adenomas (serrated adenomas) following a different sequence of genetic defect accumulation.

Location of lesion within bowel

Esophageal carcinoma
Squamous cell carcinoma usually arises in the upper and mid third of the esophagus, while adenocarcinoma arises within the lower third or at the gastroesophageal junction.

Gastric carcinoma
Adenocarcinoma can occur anywhere within the stomach, although it appears to be becoming more common at the gastroesophageal junction.

Colorectal carcinoma
Adenocarcinoma can occur at any position within the colon or rectum.

Extraintestinal manifestations

None, apart from metastases and related extracolonic conditions, as described above.

Diagnostic tests

Depending on the mode of presentation, barium contrast radiologic examination might demonstrate a stricture, while endoscopy will usually enable biopsy of a lesion for histological confirmation of its nature. Cross-sectional imaging (computed tomography or magnetic resonance imaging scanning) is almost universally used in the UK for tumor staging. Endoscopic ultrasound examination is being used increasingly frequently in the UK for the assessment and staging of esophageal tumors.

Major immunopathologic features

Esophageal carcinoma

There appears to be a causative link between gastroesophageal reflux and chronic inflammation within the lower esophagus, Barrett's esophagus, and the development of esophageal adenocarcinoma. Reflux of gastric contents and/or bile into the lower esophagus results in esophageal inflammation (esophagitis). Chronic reflux and severe associated esophagitis can predispose to replacement of a variable length of esophageal stratifed squamous epithelium by glandular mucosa (usually gastric type mucosa with a variable degree of intestinal metaplasia) – this is known as Barrett's esophagus. The glandular mucosa comprising Barrett's esophagus commonly contains acute and chronic inflammatory cells. Dysplasia of this glandular epithelium can develop in this setting and, in some cases, lead to adenocarcinoma. A similar link is not evident for squamous cell carcinoma of the esophagus, which does not develop in the setting of Barrett's esophagus.

Gastric carcinoma

Inflammatory destruction of gastric glands leads to glandular atrophy (ie, loss of glands); in the body and fundus of the stomach, this is associated with loss of the hydrochloric acid-secreting parietal cells.

Colorectal carcinoma

Most cases of colorectal carcinoma occur sporadically and are not associated with a pre-existing chronic colitis, but colorectal adenocarcinoma can develop in the setting of the chronic inflammatory mucosal damage that occurs in IBD, especially UC. Patients with IBD who possess the highest risk of carcinoma development are those in whom colitis involves the whole colon and those with longstanding colitis (ie, over 10 years duration).

Putative immunopathogenesis

Esophageal and colorectal carcinoma
The precise mechanisms linking chronic inflammation with carcinoma development within the esophagus and stomach are not known. However, longstanding inflammatory damage to the epithelium is common to carcinomas that arise in gastroesophageal reflux disease and IBD. Therefore, it seems that inflammation, when sufficiently severe and long-term, is able to induce neoplastic transformation within epithelial cells.

Gastric carcinoma
Glandular atrophy and parietal cell loss leads to hypochlorhydria and secondary bacterial overgrowth with the production of bacteria-derived carcinogens that then act on the gastric epithelial cells and result in neoplastic transformation of these cells. It is of interest that the acquired lymphoid tissue induced by *H. pylori* may also lead to the development of mucosa-associated (marginal zone) lymphoma.

Treatment

Carcinomas detected at a sufficiently early stage may be surgically resectable. Chemotherapy and/or radiotherapy can be used as an adjuvant to surgery or to provide palliation in unresectable disease. Radiotherapy alone may be the potentially curative treatment of choice in conditions such as invasive squamous cell carcinoma of the anal canal.

Celiac disease

Cause

Gluten, the constituent of cereals (wheat, barley, and rye) that gives dough its viscoelasticity and water-retaining capacity. Gluten has two major components: gliadin and glutenin. It is likely that both can cause celiac disease.

Age of onset	May present in infants ≤2 years of age after wheat, rye, or barley gluten ingestion, but the disease can present at any age. Because of improved nutrition, silent celiac disease is now relatively common, where patients have a damaged intestine, but appear healthy. The disease is lifelong.
Principal clinical features	The classic celiac patient is a wasted individual with malabsorption, iron-deficiency anemia, a swollen abdomen, and steatorrhea (high-volume, evil-smelling, pale stools). However, the presentation may be more subtle. Many patients might appear outwardly healthy, but can still be identified because of iron-deficiency anemia or a pre-existing autoimmune condition (eg, insulin-dependent diabetes mellitus or thyroiditis).
Epidemiology/genetics	The prevalence might be as high as 1 in 100 in Western Europe. Over 95% of patients have a particular tissue type (HLA-DQ2) and virtually all of the rest are HLA-DQ8 positive. This is the closest association of any disease of known etiology with a particular HLA type. The disease is allegedly less common in the USA. The concept of the celiac iceberg is now accepted, in that only a minority of patients (those with overt disease) present to clinicians, while the majority remain undiagnosed.
Association with other diseases	Now that there is a very good serologic test for celiac disease (see Diagnostic tests), screening usually identifies apparently healthy people who in fact have celiac disease, and has also led to the linkage of celiac disease with other conditions, such as autoimmune hepatitis and autoimmune thyroiditis. Patients have an increased incidence of other autoimmune diseases, such as insulin-dependent diabetes mellitus. Epilepsy with posterior cerebellar calcification has also been reported. Infertility and recurrent abortion can occur in women with untreated or silent celiac disease. There is also a high incidence of IgA deficiency. There is a small but significant risk of developing enteropathy-associated T-cell

lymphoma (EATL), a malignancy of gut IELs (see p. 96).

Location of lesion within bowel

Duodenum and upper jejunum. Affected patients might also have lymphocytic gastritis and/or lymphocytic colitis.

Extraintestinal manifestations

Include defects in tooth enamel, oral apthous ulcers, hyposplenism, and cerebral calcification. Some patients develop dermatitis herpetiformis, an inflammatory condition associated with the deposition of IgA in the skin. This condition has the same genetic association as celiac disease and is also gluten responsive.

Diagnostic tests

Nearly all celiac patients have high serum levels of antibodies to gliadin, a major protein component of gluten. In children, however, these antibodies are seen in a variety of other disorders and are not specific. Patients also have high serum levels of IgA antibodies to tissue transglutaminase (tTG), an enzyme involved in collagen cross-linking. This was previously detected by the antiendomysial antibody test on monkey esophagus (endomysium is the ground substance between cells in tissues) or umbilical cord. Commercial enzyme-linked immunoabsorbent assays (ELISAs) are now available for recombinant tTG. These have a high specificity and sensitivity in most patients, although positivity is less frequent in very young children.

It is important to ensure that a lack of IgA anti-tTG in a patient is not due to IgA deficiency. In these patients, IgG anti-tTG antibodies are present. Positive anti-tTG antibody reactivity is so specific for celiac disease that it can replace the need for small-bowel biopsy, at least in adult patients. However, upper-intestinal biopsy is still the gold standard for diagnosis, although the rigorous diagnostic criteria of earlier years (flat mucosa when untreated, resolution on a gluten-free diet, and appearance of the lesion on gluten challenge) are rarely applied because of the need for three separate small-bowel biopsies.

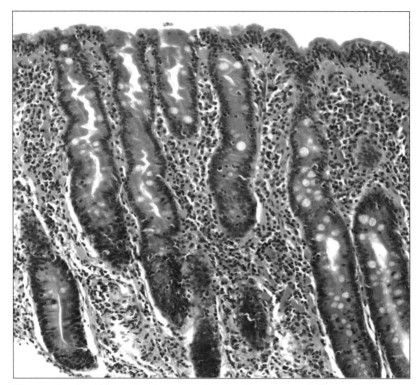

Figure 7. Duodenal biopsy showing mucosal remodeling with loss of villi, crypt hyperplasia, an increased intraepithelial lymphocyte count, and increased chronic inflammatory cell numbers within the lamina propria. The appearance is entirely consistent with that of active celiac disease.

Hematoxylin and eosin stain. Magnification ×200.

Major immunopathologic features

Duodenal or jejunal biopsy might reveal mucosal remodeling, with loss of villi and crypt hyperplasia, to give the classic "flat mucosa" (**Figure 7**).

However, many patients show partial villous atrophy and there might be only minor villous blunting. Patients also have mucosal edema. There is an increase in chronic inflammatory cell numbers in the LP, and an increase in the density of IELs. In fact, IEL numbers are not increased, but might in fact be slightly decreased in absolute terms; they only appear increased because of the dramatic reduction in villus surface, which increases lymphocyte density in relation to enterocytes.

These changes can be patchy, especially within the duodenum, so multiple good-sized biopsies will optimize the chance of a confident histologic diagnosis. A characteristic feature of celiac disease is an increased number of γδ T cells in the epithelium; in some countries, this is used to aid diagnosis.

Putative Immunopathogenesis

Celiac disease is an excellent model in which to study mucosal immunology and inflammation because, unlike most other diseases, we know the antigen (gluten) and the HLA molecule that presents the antigen to T cells (HLA-DQ). There is very little doubt that celiac disease is due to an exaggerated Th1 response in the gut LP to gluten. An increased proportion of T cells freshly isolated from biopsies make IFNγ; when these cells are cloned, they secrete Th1-type cytokines when stimulated with gluten *in vitro*.

Recent studies have clearly shown that the enzyme tTG can modify gluten peptides so that they bind more efficiently to the HLA-DQ2 or -DQ8 molecule on APC, so the peptides are more readily recognized by T cells. CD4+ T cells in the LP then recognize the peptide–DQ2 complex and release Th1-type cytokines such as IFNγ and TNFα. These cytokines then drive mucosal remodeling, whereby LP fibroblasts change the shape of the gut and transform the normal villous structure into the flat mucosa (**Figure 8**). Celiac patients typically have very high densities of IELs – while this is of diagnostic use, there is, as yet, very little evidence that IELs are involved in the lesion or recognize gluten.

An intriguing aspect of celiac disease is that although the disease is caused by gluten, the diagnostic test involves detecting an autoantibody to tTG. Everyone has tTG in his/her gut, located just below the epithelium where it presumably remodels the basement membrane, so the antibodies cannot be caused by direct exposure

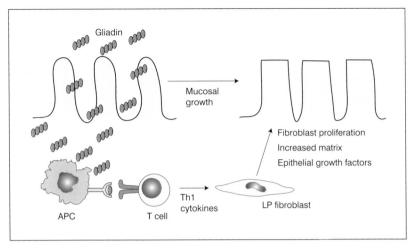

Figure 8. The mechanism of lesion formation in celiac disease. T cells in the LP respond to gliadin peptides and secrete cytokines. They change the function of LP fibroblasts, which remodel the mucosa to produce the classically flat lesion. APC: antigen-presenting cell; LP: lamina propria; Th: T-helper cell.

to the antigen. The most likely explanations for the anti-tTG antibodies are that gliadin is a substrate for tTG and that all individuals have B cells specific for self antigens, such as tTG, but which are anergic (unable to respond when they bind antigen). Gliadin–tTG complexes may form in the LP and, by a process called the carrier effect, T cells recognizing gliadin would produce cytokines and help B cells recognizing tTG to become plasma cells and secrete antibodies, breaking self tolerance (**Figure 9**).

The HLA-DQ2 haplotype is common in Western Europe (25%), so other environmental and genetic factors must be important in triggering the disease. There is very high, but not complete, concordance for celiac disease in identical twins, indicating that factors additional to genetic influences must be important.

Treatment

The vast majority of patients respond well to a gluten-free diet, although a few also require steroid therapy to induce remission. In some cases, remission can take many months, despite a strict

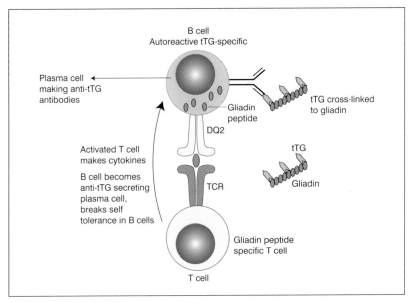

Figure 9. The immunological basis for the production of antibodies to tTG: tTG binds to gliadin. All individuals have B cells with specificity (ie, surface antibody molecules) for tTG, but the B cells are anergic. Normally, when tTG binds, the B cells would not respond. However, B cells are also potent antigen-presenting cells and take up gliadin-tTG and present gliadin peptides to T cells on DQ2 molecules. The T cell then becomes activated and produces cytokines such as interleukin-2, which are sufficient to make the anergic B cell start to divide and become a plasma cell, secreting anti-tTG antibodies. TCR: T-cell receptor; tTG: tissue transglutaminase.

gluten-free diet. Oat gluten apparently does not cause the disease, but contamination of oats with wheat gluten during milling can be a problem, as can the presence of gluten in many foods.

Chronic granulomatous disease

Cause

A genetic deficiency of phagocytic activity, leading to an inability to kill certain commonly encountered microorganisms. This results in immunodeficiency and susceptibility, particularly to bacterial and fungal infections of the respiratory tract, skin, and soft tissues (especially staphylococcae; also atypical

Mycobacterium, *Nocardia*, and *Salmonella* species). The specific defect is an inability of neutrophils and macrophages to produce superoxide anions, which kill microorganisms.

Age of onset	Infancy
Principal clinical features	Esophageal dysmotility, inflammation, and strictures, which can occur with or without demonstrable infection. Intestinal involvement can also lead to steatorrhea, vitamin B_{12} deficiency, and obstruction.
Epidemiology/genetics	X-linked (defective cytochrome B558) or autosomal recessive (defective NADPH oxidase component) inheritance.
Association with other diseases	None
Location of lesion within bowel	Small or large intestine.
Extraintestinal manifestations	Recurrent infections, multifocal abscesses of the skin and liver, lymphadenopathy, hepatosplenomegaly, chronic lung disease, and persistent diarrhea.
Diagnostic tests	The nitroblue tetrazolium test is definitive for diagnosis. Normal blood neutrophils in culture can reduce the soluble clear dye nitroblue tetrazolium to an insoluble blue precipitate, formazan, which can be clearly seen within the cells. Most patients with CGD have a complete deficiency of this ability – in some cases, however, a percentage of neutrophils may be functional.
Major immunopathologic features	Esophageal biopsy usually shows non-specific inflammation only. In the small bowel, there might be normal morphology with lipid-filled villi, but the disease often occurs as an enterocolitis similar to Crohn's disease (see p. 86). Deep fissuring ulcers can be present, with transmural inflammation and patchy lesions. Granulomas and giant cells can be seen. The mucosa is infiltrated with mononuclear cells. The similarity with Crohn's disease extends

to the development of perianal abscesses and fistulae (**Figure 10**).

Crohn's-like lesions in CGD and even rarer phagocytic deficiencies such as glycogen storage disease type 1B (see p. 101) are very informative for the pathogenesis of Crohn's disease. The gut of children with CGD does not contain a known pathogen, and so the lesion is almost certainly driven by the normal flora, abundant in the ileum and colon.

It is known that the normal flora cross the gut epithelium at a low level in healthy individuals, in a process called translocation. Phagocytes below the epithelium usually kill these microbes. However, when there is a deficiency in killing by macrophages and neutrophils, the organisms may persist as microabscesses and elicit a local Th1 response, as in Crohn's disease (**Figure 11**). Inflammation will then result in a break in the epithelial barrier, allowing the ingress of more bacteria and a continuing cycle of inflammation. The fact that a Crohn's-like lesion can occur in children with CGD does not mean that patients with Crohn's have a defect in their neutrophils. Instead, it shows that Crohn's-like pathology can occur when the immune system is dysregulated, similar to the many animal models of Crohn's disease, where many different immunologic changes can result in an identical gut pathology.

Treatment

Supportive treatment is required, ie, treatment of infections with antibiotics and surgery (eg, drainage of abscesses), as appropriate. Prophylactic antibiotics may be indicated in some patients. IFNγ therapy can reduce the frequency of infections by increasing the effectiveness of macrophage killing of microorganisms. Bone marrow transplantation is curative.

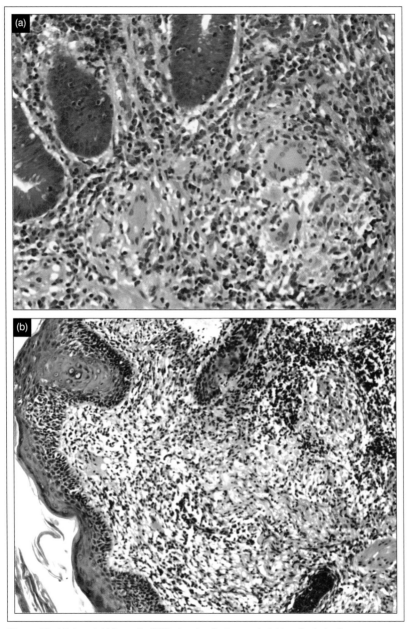

Figure 10. (a) A rectal biopsy in CGD showing features mimicking Crohn's disease, with well-formed granulomas present. (b) Perianal skin in CGD showing florid granulomatous inflammation. CGD: chronic granulomatous disease.

Hematoxylin and eosin stains. Magnification ×200.

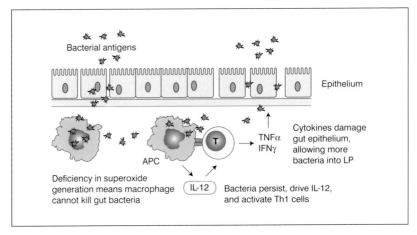

Figure 11. Putative pathogenesis of CGD. Gut bacteria constantly cross the gut epithelium at low levels. In normal individuals these are killed by subepithelial macrophages. In children with CGD, the bacteria cannot be killed and they persist in the LP. This then triggers a Th1 response through excess production of IL-12. The mucosa is damaged and a cycle of chronic inflammation ensues. Mechanistically this is very much like Crohn's disease. APC: antigen presenting cell; CGD: chronic granulomatous disease; IFN: interferon; IL: interleukin; LP: lamina propria; Th: T-helper cell; TNF: tumor necrosis factor.

Collagenous colitis

Cause	Unknown. Some cases occur in association with non-steroidal anti-inflammatory drug (NSAID) usage.
Age of onset	The peak age of onset is the sixth decade, but the disease can occur at almost any age.
Gender bias	The male to female ratio is 1:6.
Principal clinical features	Watery (not bloody) diarrhea is the principal symptom. There may be a history of several years' duration. Abdominal pain and weight loss are not uncommon.
Epidemiology/genetics	This is a rare condition. It occurs in families, which suggests a possible genetic association.
Association with other diseases	The clinical picture overlaps with that of lymphocytic colitis (see p. 111), and these diseases are believed by many to represent part of the same "microscopic

     A–Z Disease Listing

colitis" disease spectrum. There is an association with celiac disease (see p. 68), although this appears to be more strongly linked to lymphocytic colitis.

Location of lesion within bowel	Colon
Extraintestinal manifestations	Might be associated with arthropathy, including rheumatoid arthritis.
Diagnostic tests	Diagnosis is by histologic analysis of colonic biopsies, together with clinical history.
Major immunopathologic features	The colonoscopic appearance of the bowel is usually normal and diagnosis relies upon the identification of characteristic features within colonic biopsies. These comprise a thickened subepithelial collagen plate (>10 μm in thickness) and a diffuse increase in lymphocyte and plasma cell numbers within the LP. These features might be identifiable within a rectal biopsy, although some studies have suggested that subepithelial collagen plate thickening is most marked in the proximal colon (**Figure 12**).
	In contrast to Crohn's disease and UC, the epithelium is essentially normal, although IEL numbers might be slightly increased, along with denudation of the surface epithelium.
Putative immunopathogenesis	Unknown. It is possible to speculate that the increased numbers of inflammatory cells induce increased deposition of collagen by fibroblasts below the epithelium, or that there could be a problem with collagen breakdown so that, over time, collagen accumulates at this site. mRNA *in situ* hybridization reveals that collagen synthesis is increased in the subepithelial fibroblasts, and that, while levels of enzymes that break down collagen (matrix metalloproteinases [MMPs]) are also increased, there is an abundance of TIMP-1 (the natural inhibitor of MMPs), which could prevent the collagen-degrading enzyme from functioning in the extracellular environment (**Figure 13**).

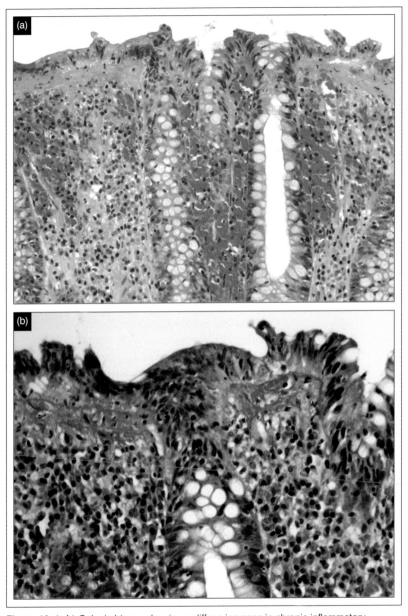

Figure 12. (a,b) Colonic biopsy showing a diffuse increase in chronic inflammatory cell numbers within the lamina propria together with thickening of the subepithelial collagen plate, characteristic of collagenous colitis.

(a) Hematoxylin and eosin stain. Magnification ×200. (b) van Giesen stain for collagen. Magnification ×400.

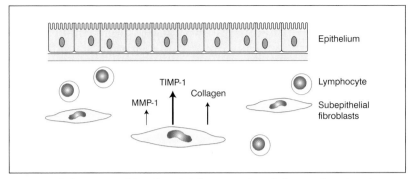

Figure 13. Collagenous colitis is the only inflammatory bowel disease where there is excess mucosal deposition of collagen. Analysis of subepithelial fibroblasts shows that they are making more collagen; however, they are also making more of the enzymes which break down collagen, so there should be no net accumulation of collagen. The amount of the natural inhibitor of MMPs, TIMP-1, is also markedly elevated. Collagenous colitis therefore might reflect the fact that excess TIMP-1 stops MMPs from breaking down collagen. MMP: matrix metalloproteinase; TIMP: tissue inhibitor of metalloproteinase.

Treatment

The disease tends to wax and wane over several years. Patients might respond to steroids or sulfasalazines. Budesonide seems particularly effective. Cholestyramine can be useful if there is concomitant bile acid malabsorption. Colectomy is seldom, but occasionally, required.

Common variable immunodeficiency

Definition

This term is used to describe a heterogeneous group of sporadic or familial Ig deficiencies, characterized by B-cell dysfunction, low levels of serum Igs, and a failure of B cells to become mature, antibody-secreting plasma cells.

Age of onset

Childhood or adult life.

Principal clinical features

Patients commonly suffer recurrent bacterial infections with recurrent otitis media, bronchopulmonary infections, diarrhea, and malabsorption. Splenomegaly might also be present.

Epidemiology/genetics	This is the second most common form of primary immunodeficiency after IgA deficiency, with an incidence of 6–12 cases per million live births.
Association with other diseases	Coexistent *Giardia* infection is present in 20%–30% of cases. Other associated infections include *Campylobacter, Shigella, Salmonella, Cryptosporidium, Cytomegalovirus,* and *Strongyloides.* Chronic atrophic gastritis occurs in 30%–50% of cases, leading to a pernicious anemia-like condition and an increased risk of gastric carcinoma. Carcinoma and lymphoma might also occur at other sites within the gastrointestinal tract.
Location of lesion within bowel	Mainly the small intestine.
Extraintestinal manifestations	Include respiratory infections and bronchiectasis.
Diagnostic tests	Duodenal or jejunal biopsy reveals histologic features that closely resemble celiac disease (see p. 68). However, plasma cells are lacking within the LP (**Figure 14**). Granulomatous inflammation may be present.
Major immunopathologic features	The disease is characterized by low levels of Igs, together with defects in CMI. The relative severity of humoral and cell-mediated deficiencies is variable. There is often an increase in the number of LP T cells and IELs. One of the most striking features is lymphonodular hyperplasia, where the mucosa contains prominent lymphoid follicles.
Putative immunopathogenesis	Deficiency in antibody production could allow more luminal antigens to enter the LP, driving a Th1 response (as in celiac disease) that causes villous blunting and crypt hyperplasia. However, the condition is not due to gluten sensitivity. Concurrent infections due to defective mucosal humoral immunity (IgA) can also cause injury.
Treatment	The mainstay of treatment is Ig replacement therapy, together with supportive treatment, eg, of infections.

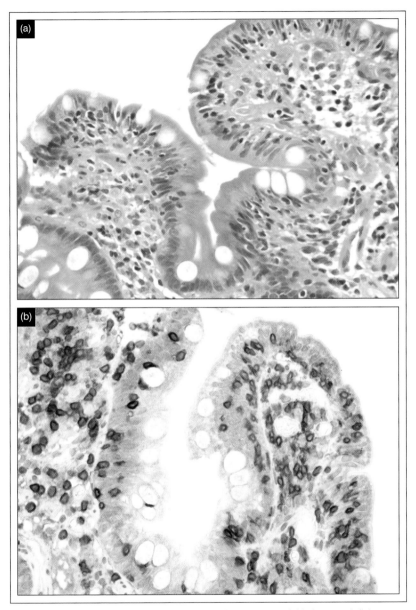

Figure 14. (**a**) Duodenal biopsy from a patient with common variable immunodeficiency, showing villous blunting and an increase in IEL numbers. The appearance can be virtually indistinguishable from that of active celiac disease. (**b**) CD3 immunohistochemistry to highlight the IELs. IEL: intraepithelial lymphocyte.

Hematoxylin and eosin stains. (**a**) Magnification ×200. (**b**) Magnification ×400.

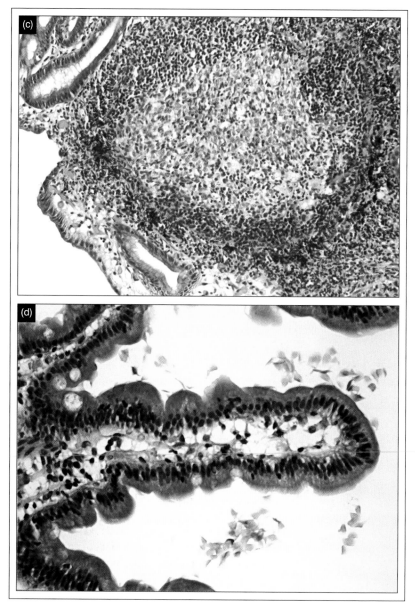

Figure 14. (continued) (c) Lymphonodular hyperplasia in a small-bowel biopsy.
(d) *Giardia* in a small-bowel biopsy.

(c,d) Hematoxylin and eosin stains. Magnification ×200.

Cows' milk-sensitive enteropathy

Cause	Cows' milk
Age of onset	Neonates and young infants.
Principal clinical features	Chronic diarrhea and failure to thrive, occasionally with constipation and vomiting.
Epidemiology/genetics	No genetic associations have been identified and, rather obviously, the disease is more common in areas where bottle-feeding is common.
Association with other diseases	The distinction between classic cows' milk allergy and cows' milk-sensitive enteropathy is rather blurred in many cases, although differences are obvious at either end of the spectrum – ie, strongly IgE-positive, skin-test-positive patients with immediate symptoms on challenge compared with IgE-negative, skin-test-negative patients with delayed onset (days). Food-sensitive enteropathy can occur after gastroenteritis, and dietary challenges are needed to distinguish between cows' milk-sensitive enteropathy and postenteritis syndrome.
Location of lesion within bowel	Upper small bowel.
Extraintestinal manifestations	None
Diagnostic tests	There is no diagnostic test. In the past, a milk exclusion diet that resulted in normalization of small-bowel biopsies, followed by challenge and deterioration of the biopsies, was considered definitive. However, this is rarely carried out because of a reluctance for multiple endoscopic examinations.
Major immunopathologic features	Small-bowel biopsy shows a patchy lesion with villus shortening and crypt hyperplasia, which can rarely resemble celiac disease (see p. 68). A major difference, however, is that, whereas in celiac disease the flat mucosa is the same thickness as the normal mucosa, in cows' milk-sensitive enteropathy

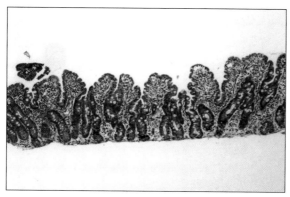

Figure 15. Duodenal biopsy from a child with cows' milk-sensitive enteropathy. There is an inflammatory infiltrate and villus blunting. Intraepithelial lymphocytes are not usually increased and the mucosa is thinner than in celiac disease.

Hematoxylin and eosin stain. Magnification ×100.

the mucosa is thinner than normal. There is an increase in LP mononuclear cell numbers, but the increase in IELs is often modest. γδ T cell levels are not increased in the epithelium (**Figure 15**).

Putative immunopathogenesis

Because of the similarity to celiac disease, cows' milk-sensitive enteropathy is thought to be due to a LP CD4 Th1 response to cows' milk proteins.

Treatment

Elimination of cows' milk from the diet and replacement with hypoallergenic formulae, such as Neocate® or Pregestimil®.

Crohn's disease

Cause

Unknown

Age of onset

The peak incidence is in young adults, with a smaller peak in the sixth and seventh decades.

Gender bias

Females are slightly more commonly affected than males.

Principal clinical features

Children and adolescents can present with failure to thrive. Abdominal pain and diarrhea, often with blood and mucus, are common (but non-specific) symptoms. Patients might present acutely with bowel obstruction, especially affecting the small bowel. The combination of non-specific abdominal pain and diarrhea, together with perianal suppurative disease (eg, perianal abscess and fistula formation), is highly suggestive of Crohn's disease.

Epidemiology/genetics

Crohn's disease affects up to 1 in 500 people in Western society. The risk of developing the disease is increased by over 30 times in first-degree relatives of affected individuals. There is also increased disease concordance in identical twins. Genome-wide scans have identified Crohn's disease susceptibility loci on chromosomes 16q12 (named *IBD1*), 12q (*IBD2*), 6p (*IBD3*), and 10. At least one of the genes responsible for susceptibility on chromosome 16 has been identified as *NOD2* (*CARD15*). The product of this gene is an intracellular bacterial-sensing molecule in macrophages. In Crohn's patients, various mutations result in a defective protein, so the mutations cause loss of function. *NOD2* mutations are probably responsible for about 15% of cases. The mutated gene on chromosome 10 is involved in maintaining epithelial integrity. Cigarette smoking is associated with a 3- to 4-fold increase in risk of disease development. There is also a profound geographic variation in the incidence of disease, as it is not commonly seen in the developing world. In the West, it is more common in individuals of higher socioeconomic status.

Association with other diseases

There is a slightly increased risk of colonic adenocarcinoma, although this risk is believed to be not as great as in UC.

Location of lesion within bowel

Any part of the gastrointestinal tract can be affected – from the mouth to the anal canal and perianal skin – but the disease is most common in the ileum (especially the terminal ileum) and colon. Fistulae may form and exteriorize on the skin, particularly following abdominal surgery, or might penetrate between adjacent loops of the gut or into other hollow viscera, such as the bladder or vagina.

Extraintestinal manifestations	Several other organs can be involved, in a similar way to UC (see p. 142). These include the liver (sclerosing cholangitis), eye (uveitis, episcleritis), skin (erythema nodosum, pyoderma gangrenosum), and joints (seronegative arthropathy). In children, Crohn's disease can lead to severe growth stunting and pubertal delay.
Diagnostic tests	Confident diagnosis is usually reliant upon a combination of clinical features, together with characteristic or supportive radiologic and histologic features. Radiologic investigations (eg, barium follow-through) might identify skip lesions, linear ulcers, apthous ulcers, fistulae, and stenoses. Histologic examination of biopsies from affected areas can reveal characteristic appearances, especially the presence of non-caseating granulomas and transmural inflammation if the biopsy includes part of the submucosa (**Figure 16**). However, the histologic features alone might not be entirely specific, and correlation with the clinical and radiologic findings is required. Patients with Crohn's disease might have raised levels of antibodies to the yeast *Saccharomyces cerevisiae* (ASCA), whereas patients with UC have raised levels of autoantibodies to neutrophil cytoplasmic proteins. By carrying out both tests, some guidance for diagnosis can be made, but definitive diagnosis is still made by histology, clinical history, and disease course. During exacerbations of the disease, serum albumin is low and the erythrocyte sedimentation rate and serum CRP concentrations are raised.
Major immunopathologic features	Inflammation of the bowel is characteristically patchy and transmural, extending deep into the gut wall. Acute and chronic inflammatory cells are abundant in the mucosa. Non-caseating granulomata are a feature of Crohn's disease and are rarely seen in UC, but are not seen in all Crohn's patients. There can be extensive fibrosis and thickening of the external muscle layers. Deep fissuring ulcers that penetrate into the submucosa are seen in severe disease.

A–Z Disease Listing

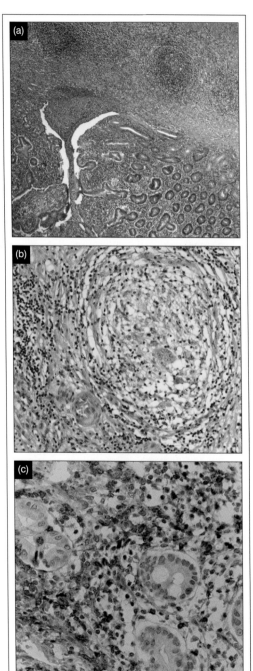

Figure 16. (a) An ileal resection specimen from a patient with Crohn's disease, showing acute and chronic inflammation within the mucosa and submucosa as a component of transmural inflammation. An area of ulceration is present. (b) A well-formed granuloma, which is typical of Crohn's disease. (c) Large numbers of CD4+ T lymphocytes are present within the lamina propria, with focal infiltration of the epithelium.

(a) Hematoxylin and eosin stain. Magnification ×50.
(b) Hematoxylin and eosin stain. Magnification ×200.
(c) CD4 immunohistochemistry. Magnification ×400.

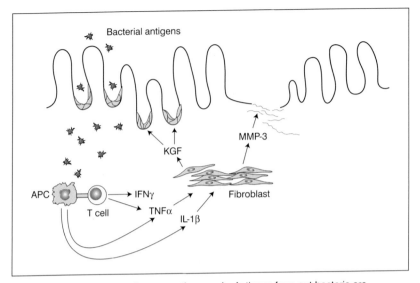

Figure 17. Crohn's disease immunopathogenesis. Antigens from gut bacteria are presented to T cells in the LP. These T cells make IFNγ and TNFα, and the IFNγ also induces macrophages to make TNFα and IL-1β. These cytokines then act on fibroblasts in the LP to produce excess MMP-3, an enzyme that breaks down the connective tissue of the mucosa and causes ulcers. At the same time, the fibroblasts produce KGF, which makes epithelial cells divide more rapidly. APC: antigen-presenting cell; IFN: interferon; IL: interleukin; KGF: keratinocyte growth factor; LP: lamina propria; MMP: matrix metalloproteinase; TNF: tumor necrosis factor.

Putative Immunopathogenesis

Crohn's disease is caused by a strong Th1 response in the LP (**Figure 17**). There is marked over-expression of T cells secreting IFNγ and TNFα, and a pronounced infiltration of TNFα- and IL-1β-secreting macrophages. The Th1-inducing cytokine IL-12 is also abundant in diseased mucosa. Increased cytokine concentrations in the mucosa up-regulate the expression of adhesion molecules on vascular endothelium so that more inflammatory cells are recruited from the blood. Cytokines also activate resident fibroblasts to secrete matrix-degrading enzymes (MMPs), which are probably responsible for ulceration. Inflammation results in the destruction of the epithelial barrier, with ingress of the luminal contents into the mucosa, and non-specific injury. This then sets up a vicious cycle of injury and repair. At the same time, mucosal fibroblasts are also producing epithelial growth factors, such as keratinocyte growth factor, which helps to produce crypt hyperplasia.

The key question is: which agent is responsible for driving the Th1 response? Although single etiological agents have been proposed, the bulk of the evidence suggests that the normal bacterial flora are crucially important. It is unlikely that a single member of the flora is responsible for the disease, but there are over 400 species of gut bacteria in great abundance in the colon and ileum, any one of which could potentially drive a Th1 response.

Studies in mice with genetically modified immune systems have conclusively shown that the normal bacterial flora can produce chronic IBD. The fact that many different changes to the immune system of mice lead to T cells reacting to the normal gut bacteria suggests that Crohn's disease is a very heterogeneous condition. This is backed up by the genetic investigations, where single gene mutations account for only a minority of patients.

Treatment

Many patients are successfully treated with corticosteroid therapy. Although effective at treating the symptoms, steroids do not heal the gut particularly well and have serious side effects. Azathioprine is highly effective, and does heal the intestine but takes weeks or months to begin to have activity. Enteral nutrition is the mainstay of treatment in pediatric Crohn's disease, but the mechanism of action is unknown. Novel therapies include monoclonal anti-TNFα therapy (infliximab), which is of proven efficacy in severe disease, especially with fistulation. Controlled trials have also shown that blocking lymphocyte migration into the gut is effective. Patients with severe disease that are unresponsive to medical treatment might require bowel resection, and surgical intervention is often required in cases of fistulation, perianal sepsis, and obstruction.

Diversion colitis

Cause	Surgical isolation of the rectum and/or colon, with diversion of the fecal stream.
Age of onset	Any
Principal clinical features	Abdominal pain, together with rectal bleeding and passage of mucus. However, the condition can also be asymptomatic.
Epidemiology/genetics	Not applicable – it is an iatrogenic disease.
Association with other diseases	Diversion colitis is particularly common after partial colectomy for UC.
Location of lesion within bowel	Defunctioned colon/rectum.
Extraintestinal manifestations	None
Diagnostic tests	The clinical history of intestinal surgery and segmental defunctioning is clearly critical, together with characteristic biopsy features (**Figure 18**).
Major immunopathologic features	Endoscopy reveals typical features of a colitis/proctitis, such as erythema, petechial hemorrhages, mucosal friability, and apthous ulcers. Mucosal biopsy of diverted normal colon shows mucosal inflammation, with foci of acute inflammation, cryptitis, crypt abscesses, and mucus depletion. Granulomas may be seen near ruptured crypts. These features can lead to an erroneous diagnosis of IBD after surgery for other conditions, or of Crohn's disease after surgery for UC. Therefore, if doubt exists regarding the original disease process, review of the originally resected bowel histology is essential. Prominent mucosal lymphoid follicles are a typical feature of diversion colitis, especially in children.
Putative immunopathogenesis	Unknown. The diverted bowel does not receive luminal nutrients so there will be changes in the normal flora and deficiency in short-chain fatty

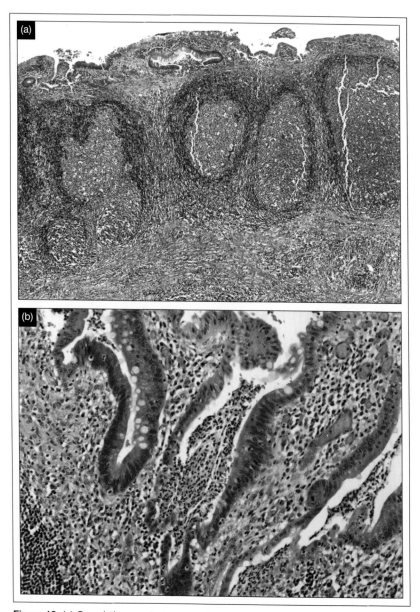

Figure 18. (a) Completion proctectomy specimen showing the features of diversion proctitis. Marked chronic inflammation is present, with prominent lymphoid aggregate and germinal center formation. (b) A higher-power view of the mucosa to show acute inflammation, with neutrophil infiltration of the surface epithelium and associated surface acute inflammatory debris.

Hematoxylin and eosin stains. (a) Magnification ×50. (b) Magnification ×200.

acids. These are made from fiber by the gut bacteria, and are a major energy substrate for colonic epithelial cells. Butyrate (a short-chain fatty acid) has been instilled into the defunctioned bowel to restore short-chain fatty acids, but the clinical response is inconsistent.

Treatment	Surgical reversal of the defunctioned segment leads to a prompt clinical response.

Enterobiasis

Cause	Infection with the nematode *Enterobius vermicularis*.
Age of onset	Children are the most commonly affected.
Principal clinical features	Perianal itching and pain are common. Appendiceal involvement may be associated with the development of acute appendicitis. Heavy infection can lead to the development of fibrous nodules within the bowel mucosa and bowel obstruction. The worm can produce perianal abscesses and invade the peritoneal cavity via the female reproductive system, causing pelvic peritonitis.
Epidemiology/genetics	Worldwide distribution
Association with other diseases	None
Location of lesion within bowel	The larvae hatch within the small intestine and mate within the large intestine. The eggs are then carried to the anus. Autoinfection commonly occurs, with transmission of eggs to the mouth on the child's fingers. Alternatively, the eggs can hatch on the perianal skin, with larvae migrating back into the rectum.
Extraintestinal manifestations	In rare cases, the worm can disseminate to the liver and cause granulomata.

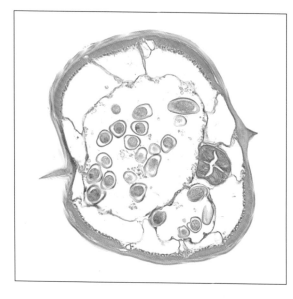

Figure 19. Transverse section of an *Enterobius vermicularis* worm showing the characteristic lateral spines.
Hematoxylin and eosin stain. Magnification ×200.

Diagnostic tests

Diagnosis relies upon identification of worms with the characteristic morphology in stool samples or biopsy specimens (especially appendicectomy specimens) (**Figure 19**). Clear adhesive tape applied to the anus can be examined microscopically for the presence of eggs.

Major immunopathologic features

There is an increase in eosinophil numbers in the mucosa. Granulomatous mucosal inflammation occasionally occurs.

Putative immunopathogenesis

Parasitic worms classically elicit Th2 responses (IgE, eosinophils, and mast cells infiltrate into tissues), but much of the perianal damage is undoubtedly due to scratching.

Treatment

Proper hygiene is essential, due to the high risk of autoinfection as described above, or transmission on clothes or bed linen. Mebendazole or piperazine therapy should eradicate the parasites.

Enteropathy-associated T-cell lymphoma

Cause	A lymphoma associated with celiac disease.
Age of onset	Late to middle age.
Principal clinical features	The most common local effect is small intestinal obstruction or perforation. Patients can also present with typical celiac disease symptoms of malabsorption and anemia, which do not respond to gluten withdrawal.
Epidemiology/genetics	These are essentially the same as for celiac disease (see p. 68). HLA genotypes (DQ2/DQ8) associated with subclinical or delayed-clinical-onset celiac disease confer a higher risk of development of EATL, possibly due to long-term, low-grade stimulation of the gut immune system by gluten. EATL is almost certainly related to refractory sprue, a celiac-like, gluten-insensitive enteropathy that contains clonal populations of T cells and that may be cryptic EATL (see p. 134).
Association with other diseases	Patients usually have a history of celiac disease. In these cases, histologic features of celiac disease are often present within the adjacent non-neoplastic small-bowel mucosa.
Location of lesion within bowel	Small bowel, but tumor cells are present along the length of the gut.
Extraintestinal manifestations	None, apart from dissemination of the lymphoma.
Diagnostic tests	Radiologic examination or surgical exploration might reveal one or multiple small-bowel lesions. Histologic examination of biopsy or resection material reveals a T-cell non-Hodgkin's lymphoma, which is most commonly high grade in nature (**Figure 20**).
Major immunopathologic features	The appearance of the mucosa resembles the flat lesion of celiac disease. However, ulcers may be present and there is a massive infiltrate of clonal

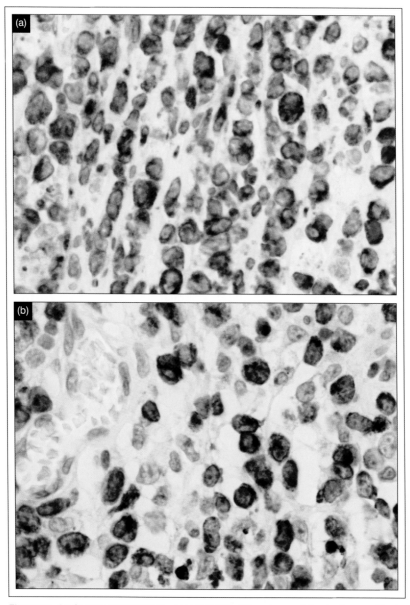

Figure 20. (a) Section of enteropathy-associated T-cell lymphoma stained with an antibody to CD3. The tumor contains large numbers of positive cells, but they are unusual in that CD3 is in the cytoplasm and not the membrane. **(b)** The malignant T cells express markers associated with cytotoxic T cells, in this case, perforin.

(a,b) Immunoperoxidase. Magnification ×400.

lymphocytes (all derived from the same single malignant precursor). The phenotype of the tumor cells is highly unusual in that in most patients they are clearly T cells since they have a rearranged TCRγ chain, but they are often CD4, CD8, and TCR negative, yet express cytoplasmic CD3. In some cases the tumor cells express CD8. The tumor cells express the CD103 integrin (αEβ7) that is found on IELs, which suggests that the tumor itself is derived from IELs. Many patients with refractory sprue also have clonal populations of these unusual IELs.

Putative immunopathogenesis	The genomic changes in EATL remain unknown. The flat lesion in these patients is thought to be driven by malignant IELs, but few functional studies have yet been carried out on these cells. Tumor cells appear to be dependent on a cytokine (IL-15) for growth. IL-15 is made by many cell types and is thought to be a factor that stops T cells from undergoing apoptosis (programmed cell death). EATL is a rare condition, and fresh cells or frozen material are rarely available for study.
Treatment	Surgical resection combined with chemotherapy. The prognosis of this aggressive malignancy is usually poor.

Eosinophilic gastroenteritis

Cause	Unknown
Age of onset	Most commonly between the second and third decades.
Gender bias	The male to female ratio is 2:1.
Principal clinical features	Bloating and vomiting soon after eating certain foods, although, in some cases, disease is not associated with a specific food. Growth failure might occur. Colonic disease results in episodic

abdominal pain and diarrhea. Involvement of the intestinal serosa (the least common pattern) can result in recurrent eosinophilic ascites. Dyspepsia might also occur.

Epidemiology/genetics	Rare. There are no known genetic associations.
Association with other diseases	Some patients also suffer from connective tissue diseases. There might be a history of atopy (eg, asthma, eczema) or urticaria. About 50% of patients have no history of atopy and the disease does not respond to dietary manipulation. Some patients have raised IgE levels.
Location of lesion within bowel	The disease can affect the stomach, small intestine, or colon, but most commonly involves the distal stomach.
Extraintestinal manifestations	None
Diagnostic tests	The clinical history could suggest an allergic etiology. Between 70% and 100% of patients possess an elevated peripheral blood eosinophil count. Diagnosis of the serosal form of the disease requires cytologic examination of ascitic fluid.
Major immunopathologic features	Mucosal and submucosal disease might be identified by edema on endoscopy and confirmed on biopsy histology, with submucosal edema, elevated tissue eosinophil numbers, and infiltration of crypt epithelium by eosinophils (**Figure 21**).
Putative immunopathogenesis	In individuals with a history of atopy and elevated IgE, the eosinophilia is almost certainly caused by a Th2 response, since IL-5 made by Th2 cells is a potent eosinophil growth factor. In patients with no history of atopy, the cause is unknown.
Treatment	Avoidance of foods identified as causative agents is the first line of treatment. Oral disodium cromoglycate or alternate-day steroid therapy might be required in more severe cases.

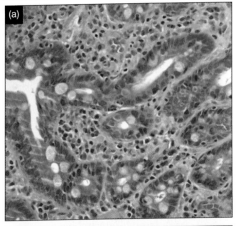

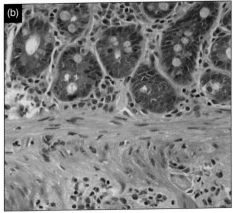

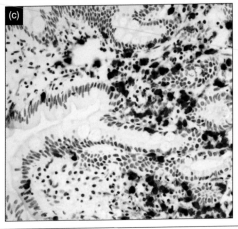

Figure 21. (a) Duodenal biopsy from a patient with eosinophilic enteritis, showing increased numbers of eosinophils within the lamina propria with focal eosinophilic infiltration of crypt epithelium.
(b) Submucosa from the same biopsy, showing characteristic eosinophilic infiltration.
(c) Immunohistochemical staining for EG2 (antibody against an eosinophil protein) to highlight the eosinophils within the mucosa.

(a–c) Hematoxylin and eosin stains. Magnification ×400.

Giardiasis

Cause	The protozoan *Giardia lamblia*.
Age of onset	Any age, but more common in children.
Principal clinical features	Infection can be asymptomatic, but common symptoms include abdominal pain, bloating, and malabsorption.
Epidemiology/genetics	The organism has a worldwide distribution, but is more common in the tropics. Infection can occur via drinking water or through the fecal–oral route.
Association with other diseases	Immunodeficiency states, especially selective IgA deficiency and common variable immunodeficiency, are associated with a significantly increased risk of giardiasis.
Location of lesion within bowel	The infection is primarily sited within the duodenum and jejunum, although small numbers of organisms may also be found within the stomach.
Extraintestinal manifestations	None
Diagnostic tests	Diagnosis relies on identification of the organisms within a stool sample (cysts or trophozoites) or small intestinal biopsy (trophozoites) (**Figure 22**). An ELISA test is available to measure *Giardia* antibodies in serum.
Major immunopathologic features	Biopsy might reveal a variable degree of villous blunting that mimics celiac disease (see p. 68), but many patients have normal mucosal morphology. Epithelial γδ T cell numbers are not elevated. Trophozoites can be seen closely associated with epithelium.
Putative immunopathogenesis	The resemblance to celiac disease suggests that, in patients with villus atrophy, the lesion might be driven by a Th1 response to *Giardia*; however, this has not been studied in humans. Villous atrophy associated with infection does not occur in T-cell-deficient mice, again supporting a role for T-cell-mediated injury.

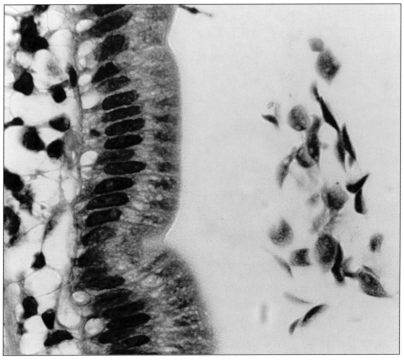

Figure 22. Duodenal biopsy showing several *Giardia* trophozoites adjacent to a villus. Giemsa stain. Magnification ×1,000.

Treatment	Medical treatments include metronidazole, timidazole, and mepacrine hydrochloride.

Glycogen storage disease type 1b

Cause	This is a rare, autosomal recessive, inborn error of metabolism caused by deficiency in gluconeogenesis. It is due to a defect in the glucose-6-phosphatase transporter, so that glucose cannot be made from glycogen, lactate, or amino acids.
Age of onset	Early infancy

Principal clinical features	Hypoglycemia, massive hepatomegaly, and growth failure. Recurrent infections occur due to defective neutrophil function, leading to abscesses, periodontal disease, and mouth ulcers.
Epidemiology/genetics	Rare, autosomal recessive
Association with other diseases	None, other than the complications of the gene defect.
Location of lesion within bowel	Type I glycogen storage disease usually affects the intestine much later in childhood. Intestinal disease usually presents as a colitis that mimics IBD.
Extraintestinal manifestations	Type I glycogen storage disease is associated with hyperuricemia and gout, since glucose-6-phosphatase deficiency interferes with the renal excretion of uric acid. Patients also suffer from hepatomegaly, growth retardation, osteopenia, kidney enlargement, hypoglycemia, hyperlactacidemia, hyperlipidemia, and neutropenia.
Diagnostic tests	Functional enzyme assay for glucose-6-phosphatase in liver homogenates.
Major immunopathologic features	The intestinal lesions in these children resemble those of Crohn's disease (see p. 86). There is transmural inflammation.
Putative immunopathogenesis	The key to the IBD in these children lies in the defective neutrophil function, since colitis is also seen in CGD (see p. 74). Neutrophils probably play a role in eliminating the low numbers of normal flora that cross the gut epithelium in all individuals. In their absence, bacteria persist and drive a Th1 response, as in Crohn's disease. However, it is not known why these children develop neutropenia.
Treatment	Successful treatment of hypoglycemia in type I glycogen storage disease can result in a good prognosis. Treatment with granulocyte colony-stimulating factor can boost neutrophil numbers, reduce infections, and help to resolve colitis. Antibiotics can also be useful in treating infections.

Graft-versus-host disease

Cause	T cells in allogeneic transplanted bone marrow reacting against the cells and tissues of the recipient, which they see as foreign.
Age of onset	Any, the disease is iatrogenic. Acute graft-versus-host disease (GVHD) disease occurs 2–10 weeks after transplantation; chronic GVHD occurs 3–12 months after transplantation.
Principal clinical features	In acute GVHD, the patient may be febrile and have a rash, which can range from mild maculopapular eruption to diffuse erythroderma. In chronic GVHD, skin lesions present as pigmentation and scleroderma-like involvement. Organ dysfunction can occur (eg, hepatitis, diarrhea).
Epidemiology/genetics	GVHD occurs in up to 40% of allogeneic bone marrow recipients.
Association with other diseases	Not applicable.
Location of lesion within bowel	In acute GVHD, the main targets are the colon and distal ileum. This leads to diarrhea, malabsorption, abdominal pain, and protein-losing enteropathy, resulting in severe gastroenteritis. Oral mucositis and polyserositis often occur in chronic GVHD. A major target is also the esophagus, which can result in dysphagia.
Extraintestinal manifestations	As well as the skin, the liver is a major target in GVHD. In acute disease, cholestasis, panlobular hepatocellular damage, and degeneration of the small bile ducts can be seen. Without immunosuppressive therapy, the disease can progress to fibrosis, portal hypertension, and liver failure. Patients with chronic GVHD might have chronic liver disease with "vanishing bile duct syndrome".
Diagnostic tests	GVHD can be a problem in all mismatched bone marrow transplants, and there is a very high awareness of the condition in specialist units.

Major immunopathologic features	Gastrointestinal mucosal biopsy reveals acute and chronic inflammation, together with epithelial cell apoptosis (a cardinal feature), especially at the base of crypts (acute GVHD) (**Figure 23**). Disease progression leads to glandular loss, ulceration, and mucosal/ submucosal fibrosis (chronic GVHD). The mucosa becomes infiltrated with T cells.
Putative Immunopathogenesis	The disease is due to T cells in the grafted marrow recognizing the recipient's cells as foreign antigens. Both CD4 and CD8 cells become activated, especially in tissues where there is high expression of MHC class II molecules, such as the gut and biliary tree. Cytotoxic T cells may kill recipient cells and CD4 cells release Th1-type proinflammatory cytokines. Recent data from mouse models have suggested that alloreactive T cells lodge and respond to the host at PPs before migrating to systemic tissues. This might also explain why the gut is a primary target.
Treatment	Immunosuppression (eg, steroids, cyclosporin) is given to reduce the incidence of both GVHD and graft rejection. Allogeneic bone marrow transplants are associated with a lower incidence of GVHD than those using matched, unrelated donors. T-cell depletion of bone marrow grafts may reduce the chance of GVHD. However, in bone marrow transplants performed for leukemia, GVHD is associated with a "graft-versus-leukemia" effect, which reduces the incidence of leukemia recurrence.

Helicobacter-associated gastritis

Cause	Colonization of the stomach by *Helicobacter pylori*. *H. heilmannii* has recently been recognized as an alternative, but far less common, causative agent, with a very similar resultant disease spectrum.
Age of onset	Any

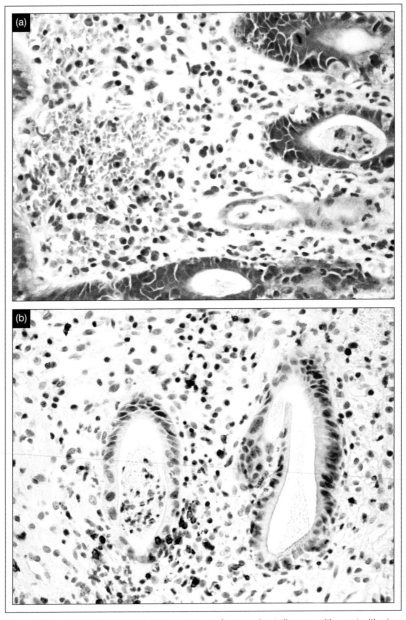

Figure 23. (a,b) Colonic biopsy showing acute graft-versus-host disease, with crypt withering associated with degenerative epithelial changes, including epithelial cell apoptosis.

(a) Hematoxylin and eosin stain. (b) Immunohistochemical staining for CD4 T cells. Magnification ×400.

Principal clinical features	Asymptomatic or associated with the development of acute or chronic gastritis, often with gastric or duodenal ulceration.
Epidemiology/genetics	*H. pylori* has a worldwide distribution. Infection can occur in childhood, particularly when social circumstances result in crowded living conditions, and infection is endemic in the tropics. The incidence increases with increasing age. Approximately 50% of 50-year-olds are infected, but infection rates are decreasing as people grow up in cleaner environments where there is less chance of infection.
Association with other diseases	*H. pylori* infection has been postulated to be associated with atherosclerosis and other systemic conditions, but this is controversial. Its role in gastroesophageal reflux disease is also not known. It is undoubtedly associated with peptic and duodenal ulcers, where it colonizes metaplastic gastric epithelium in the duodenum. The most serious associations are with lymphoma (marginal zone lymphoma; see p. 114) and adenocarcinoma of the stomach (see p. 63). Lymphoma occurs due to chronic stimulation of the immune system, leading to neoplastic transformation within acquired lymphoid tissue of the gastric mucosa. Adenocarcinoma occurs due to chronic mucosal damage, leading to intestinal metaplasia, mucosal atrophy, and secondary bacterial overgrowth, with production of carcinogenic bacterial metabolites and resultant neoplastic transformation of the gastric epithelium.
Location of lesion within bowel	The stomach is by far the most common site of *H. pylori* colonization, although the bacteria can also be found within gastric-type glandular mucosa in Barrett's esophagus and associated with surface gastric epithelial metaplasia of the duodenum in "peptic" duodenitis.

Extraintestinal manifestations	No definite association with diseases outside of the bowel has been proven with *Helicobacter* colonization, although a link has recently been suggested with coronary artery atherosclerosis.
Diagnostic tests	The presence of *Helicobacter* within the stomach can be confirmed using tests relying on bacterial urease production. These include the non-invasive carbon-13 or carbon-14 breath test, and pH indicator-based tests for fresh gastric biopsies (eg, the CLOtest®). The bacteria are usually readily identified within gastric biopsy material, and immunohistochemical staining is now available for cases in which only a small number of bacteria are present. Affected patients usually possess circulating anti-*Helicobacter* antibodies, which persist for up to a year after bacterial eradication.
Major immunopathologic features	*H. pylori* infection in children is associated with the development of acquired mucosa-associated lymphoid tissue that is similar to PPs in the gastric wall. Gastritis can be seen histologically as acute, with neutrophils in the epithelium and LP, or chronic, with a predominant lymphocyte and plasma cell infiltrate (**Figure 24**). Atrophy of the mucosa (loss of gastric glands) also occurs. *H. pylori* infection is always associated with gastritis. In adults, it is most commonly seen as an acute gastritis, whereas chronic gastritis is more common in children and significant gastric atrophy is not seen. Immunohistology has revealed an increase in epithelial T cells, LP T cells, and plasma cells in *H. pylori* infection. The infiltrating T cells have a Th1 cytokine profile.
Putative immunopathogenesis	*H. pylori* has developed numerous mechanisms to allow it to live in the acidic stomach. The principal of these is its ability to use urea as an energy substrate through the production of urease. The catalysis of urea breakdown produces ammonia, which neutralizes the stomach acid.

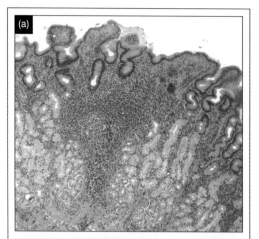

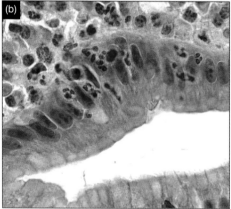

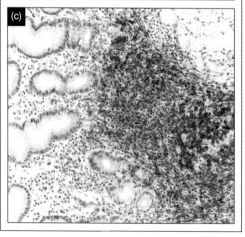

Figure 24. (a) Gastric antral biopsy, showing gastritis with lymphoid follicle formation characteristic of *Helicobacter pylori*-associated gastritis. (b) High-power view to illustrate neutrophil infiltration of the gastric foveolar epithelium. (c) Immunohistochemical staining using the B-lymphocyte marker CD20 to highlight the lymphoid aggregate.

Hematoxylin and eosin stains.
(a) Magnification ×100.
(b) Magnification ×1,000.
(c) Magnification ×200.

Although *H. pylori* is always associated with gastritis, it only rarely causes clinical disease. In addition, although there is clearly a vigorous antibacterial T-cell and antibody response, this is ineffective at eliminating the organism. Inflammation is probably due to a combination of the host antibacterial response and bacterial factors themselves. Thus, when the organism comes into contact with epithelial cells, there is a rapid release of IL-8, which attracts neutrophils into the tissue (**Figure 25**). However, because the organism lives on the gastric surface, neutrophil killing cannot occur. The neutrophils themselves, however, will damage the gastric mucosa.

The organism also produces cytotoxins such as a vacuolating toxin A (VacA), which causes epithelial cells to secrete ions and loosens epithelial tight junctions, allowing serum proteins to leak through the mucosa, which the bacteria can then use as an energy source. VacA also induces epithelial cells to undergo apoptosis and inhibits T-cell responses. The bacteria also inject proteins into epithelial cells using proteins encoded by the CAG island in their genome. The proteins injected into the host epithelial cells change the adhesion and migration properties of the epithelial cells. Strains possessing the cytotoxin-associated antigen A (*cagA*) gene are associated with increased risk of gastric cancer and peptic ulcer disease.

Animal experiments have shown that infection of mice with *H. felis* or *H. pylori* does not cause pathology in T-cell deficient mice, but that immune reconstitution of the mice and the appearance of a Th1 response in the stomach results in gastritis. This clearly suggests that some of the damage is Th1 immune mediated. Th1 clones can be grown from gastric biopsies of *H. pylori*-infected patients. There may be some similarity between the development of ulcers in *H. pylori* infection and the development of ulcers in Crohn's disease (see p. 86). In both conditions, the ulcers are

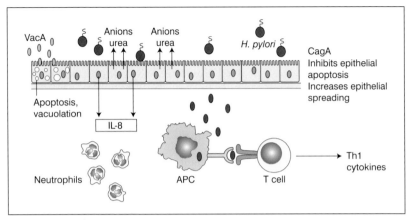

Figure 25. *Helicobacter pylori* is uniquely adapted to live in the stomach. It produces urease that catalyses urea into ammonia, which, in turn, neutralizes acid. When it binds to epithelial cells, they release IL-8, which attracts neutrophils into the mucosa. VacA secreted by the organism causes vacuolation and changes in epithelial permeability, allowing ions, urea, and plasma proteins to leak into the lumen. Using proteins encoded by the CAG pathogenicity island, *H. pylori* injects molecules into epithelial cells. These stop epithelial apoptosis and increase epithelial spreading. *H. pylori* also induces a Th1 immune response, the significance of which is unclear. APC: antigen-presenting cell; CagA: cytotoxin-associated antigen A; IL: interleukin; Th: T-helper cell; VacA: vacuolating toxin A.

surrounded by fibroblasts secreting matrix-degrading enzymes (MMPs), probably activated as a result of the local Th1 immune response.

Treatment

The antibiotics amoxicillin and clarithromycin, and a proton pump inhibitor, are the recommended treatments to eliminate the organism from the stomach.

Lymphocytic colitis

Cause

Unknown

Age of onset

Most common in the fourth and fifth decades, similar to collagenous colitis.

Principal clinical features

Profuse watery diarrhea

Epidemiology/genetics	Rare. Familial clusters have been reported, suggesting a genetic basis for the disease.
Association with other diseases	The major associations are with celiac disease and lymphocytic gastritis. The clinical picture overlaps with that of collagenous colitis (see p. 78), and these diseases are believed by many to represent part of the same "microscopic colitis" disease spectrum.
Location of lesion within bowel	Colon
Extraintestinal manifestations	Similar to collagenous colitis, in that the most common associations are with arthropathy and rheumatoid arthritis. There may also be an association with diabetes mellitus (especially insulin-dependent) and NSAID usage.
Diagnostic tests	The colonoscopic appearance of the bowel is normal, and diagnosis relies upon identification of characteristic features within colonic biopsies (**Figure 26**).
Major immunopathologic features	A diffuse increase in lymphocyte and plasma cell numbers within the LP, an increase in IEL numbers within surface and crypt epithelium, and degeneration of the surface epithelium. These features can have a patchy distribution within the colon, and examination of multiple biopsies might be required for confident diagnosis.
Putative immunopathogenesis	Unknown
Treatment	The disease tends to wax and wane over several years. Patients may respond to sulfasalazines. Non-specific antidiarrheal agents such as loperamide hydrochloride, diphenoxylate hydrochloride, and atropine or codeine are effective in some patients. Antibacterial agents such as bismuth subsalicylate, metronidazole, and erythromycin have also been effective. It is important to exclude coexistent celiac disease.

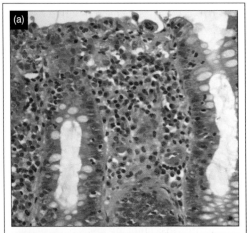

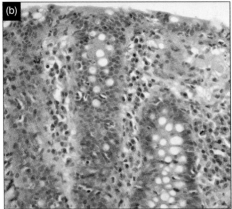

Figure 26. (a) Rectal mucosal biopsy from a patient with lymphocytic colitis showing a diffuse increase in chronic inflammatory cell numbers within the lamina propria, together with lymphocytic infiltration of the surface and crypt epithelium. The glandular architecture is preserved. (b) Connective tissue stain illustrating that the subepithelial collagen plate is of normal thickness. (c) High-power view using immunohistochemistry for T lymphocytes to highlight lymphocytic infiltration of the epithelium.

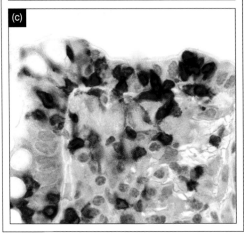

(a) Hematoxylin and eosin stain. Magnification ×400.
(b) Hematoxylin van Gieson stain. Magnification ×400.
(c) CD3 immunohistochemistry. Magnification ×1,000.

Marginal zone lymphoma

Cause	Neoplastic transformation of mucosa-associated lymphoid tissue.
Age of onset	Usually middle to old age.
Principal clinical features	These depend upon the site of the tumor. Lymphoma may present when localized to its site of origin, due to mucosal ulceration and consequent gastrointestinal hemorrhage or due to bowel obstruction. Lymphoma can also occur as an essentially incidental finding within a mucosal biopsy taken, for example, to assess endoscopically evident gastritis. Disseminated disease can present with these features, together with "general" symptoms of systemic malignancy, such as anorexia, malaise, and weight loss.
Epidemiology/genetics	Rare. The disease has a worldwide distribution, but is most common in populations with a high prevalence of *Helicobacter pylori* infection. About 90% of patients with mucosa-associated lymphoma have concomitant *H. pylori* infection.
Association with other diseases	Gastric marginal zone lymphoma is strongly associated with *H. pylori* gastritis, and appears to develop following chronic antigenic stimulation of acquired gastric lymphoid tissue, leading to neoplastic transformation. Marginal zone lymphomas arising at other sites within the gut presumably occur due to neoplastic transformation of pre-existing benign reactive lymphoid tissue.
Location of lesion within bowel	Stomach, although the small intestine and colon can also be affected.
Extraintestinal manifestations	There are none unless dissemination of the lymphoma occurs.
Diagnostic tests	Endoscopy might reveal a detectable mass that may ulcerate the mucosa. Diagnosis is made histologically. Confirmation of clonality can be achieved via polymerase chain reaction-based detection of a clonal rearrangement within one of the Ig heavy-

chain genes or by immunohistochemistry using antibodies to light chains, since each individual B cell expresses either κ or γ light chains; the presence of large numbers of either is highly suggestive of clonal expansion.

Major immunopathologic features

Diagnosis is reliant upon the identification of a neoplastic clone of lymphoid cells within biopsy material. The neoplastic cells grow in sheets, with low-grade tumors comprising centrocyte-like cells showing variable plasmacytic differentiation, colonizing pre-existing lymphoid follicles, and infiltrating glandular epithelium with a characteristic pattern ("lymphoepithelial lesions") (**Figure 27**). High-grade tumors show fewer of these characteristics and can be difficult to classify as marginal zone lymphomas unless a coexistent low-grade component is present.

Putative immunopathogenesis

The malignant B cells in gastric lymphoma show specificity for autoantigens and not for *H. pylori*. However, tumor-infiltrating T cells do respond to *H. pylori* antigens and secrete Th1 cytokines. It is therefore thought that the relatively, often non-progressive, benign nature of the tumor is because the B cells are proliferating due to local T-cell help. Tumors that do not respond to *H. pylori* have a characteristic chromosome 11;18 translocation. In contrast, malignant clones without this translocation respond well to *H. pylori* eradication.

Treatment

Despite showing morphologic and molecular biological features of neoplasia, gastric marginal cell lymphomas may regress, at least within their early stages, after *H. pylori* eradication. Tumors that are unresponsive to this treatment require conventional chemotherapy. Both low-grade and a proportion of high-grade marginal zone lymphomas remain localized to their site of origin for a relatively long period, and might therefore also be amenable to surgical therapy.

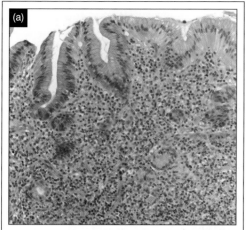

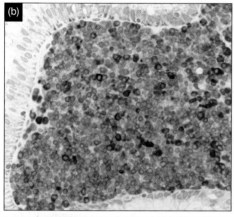

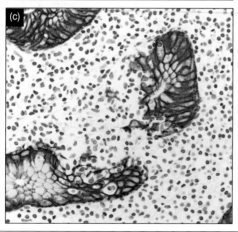

Figure 27. (**a**) Gastric mucosal biopsy from a patient with marginal zone lymphoma, showing an intense diffuse infiltrate of neoplastic lymphocytes within the lamina propria.
(**b**) Immunohistochemistry using the B-lymphocyte marker CD79a, demonstrating that the neoplastic cells are B lymphocytes.
(**c**) Immunohistochemistry using the epithelial marker cytokeratin (CAM 5.2) to highlight residual gastric glands, which contain "lymphoepithelial lesions" characteristic of marginal cell lymphoma.

Hematoxylin and eosin stains.
(**a**) Magnification ×200.
(**b**) Magnification ×400.
(**c**) Magnification ×400.

Mastocytosis

Cause	Increased numbers of mast cells, either limited to the skin or present within multiple organs.
Age of onset	Cutaneous disease usually presents in childhood, with resolution in most cases. Systemic disease usually develops in adult life.
Principal clinical features	The most common presentation is urticaria pigmentosa due to skin involvement. Localized aggregates of mast cells can produce clinical masses (mastocytomas). In systemic disease, gastrointestinal presentations include nausea, vomiting, watery diarrhea, abdominal pain, malabsorption, peptic ulceration, and, occasionally, gastrointestinal bleeds. Other features of systemic disease include headaches, bronchospasm, and hepatosplenomegaly.
Epidemiology/genetics	At least some cases are due to mutations in the molecules that control mast cell growth and development from bone marrow precursors into mature mast cells. Stem cell factor is produced by fibroblasts, endothelial cells, and marrow stromal cells. It acts on pluripotent hematopoietic stem cells and orchestrates the growth and differentiation of mast cells. Its receptor on mast cells is c-KIT. Some patients with mastocytosis have activating mutations of c-KIT so that the receptor is constantly switched on and delivers a signal to the cell to keep dividing.
Association with other diseases	None
Location of lesion within bowel	Small intestine
Extraintestinal manifestations	Systemic mastocytosis also involves the skin, bones, lungs, liver, spleen, and lymph nodes.
Diagnostic tests	Histology and clinical presentation. A commercial ELISA is available to measure serum tryptase derived from mast cells: elevated serum concentrations of >20 ng/mL identify patients more likely to have mastocytosis.

Major immunopathologic features	Small-bowel biopsy reveals increased mast cell numbers within the LP, extending into the glands, as well as within the muscularis mucosa and submucosa. Increased eosinophil numbers may also be present in association with this mast cell infiltrate.
Putative immunopathogenesis	The disease is caused by the release of mediators from the increased numbers of mast cells in the tissues. There are three main types of mediator:

- Preformed secretory granule mediators such as histamine cause pruritis, gastric hypersecretion, and increased vascular permeability.

- Lipid-derived mediators such as leukotrienes and prostaglandins cause vasoconstriction and increased vascular permeability.

- Proinflammatory cytokines such as TNFα cause cachexia and increase vascular adhesion molecule expression, and transforming growth factor-β causes fibrosis.

Treatment	Treatment is mainly symptomatic and even those with systemic disease have a good prognosis. Antihistamines can control pruritis and H-2 antagonists can control excess gastric acid secretion. Disodium cromoglycate relieves general complaints of muscle pain, headaches, and skin symptoms in some patients.

Neonatal necrotizing enterocolitis

Cause	Massive necrosis of the gut wall.
Age of onset	Premature neonates, usually of <30 weeks' gestation, within the first 3 weeks of life.
Principal clinical features	Vomiting, abdominal distension, and the appearance of blood and mucus in the stools.

Epidemiology/genetics	Approximately 6% of premature neonates. Neonatal necrotizing enterocolitis (NEC) is much more common in formula-fed infants.
Association with other diseases	Other diseases associated with prematurity may coexist with NEC (eg, intraventricular hemorrhage).
Location of lesion within bowel	The small intestine or colon, with the terminal ileum and proximal colon most commonly affected.
Extraintestinal manifestations	Disseminated intravascular coagulation can occur. The release of bacterial endotoxins into the portal circulation can result in the impairment of hepatic function and later develop to septic shock. Without intervention, NEC has a very high mortality rate.
Diagnostic tests	Abdominal X-ray reveals a thickened bowel wall containing intramural gas.
Major immunopathologic features	Resected affected bowel is dilated and necrotic. Histologic examination reveals mucosal and often transmural necrosis, with large numbers of macrophages and neutrophils present within the bowel wall (**Figure 28**).
Putative immunopathogenesis	Prematurity associated with fetal asphyxia and a reduced capacity for the neonatal intestine to take up oxygen, especially during periods of feeding, might lead to mucosal ischemia and translocation of bacteria, with associated toxins, from the lumen into the wall of the gut (**Figure 29**). The lesion contains few T cells so the damage is due to non-specific effector cells, probably responding to components of the flora. TNFα and platelet-activating factor (PAF) concentrations are high in the diseased bowel. There is also a marked increase in fibroblast-derived, matrix-degrading enzymes (MMPs), probably as a result of the increased local TNFα.
	Injection of TNFα, LPS, or PAF into the circulation of baby rats produces rapid necrosis of the bowel, suggesting that these mediators, which have been identified in the gut and serum of infants with NEC, may be primarily involved in driving the lesions.

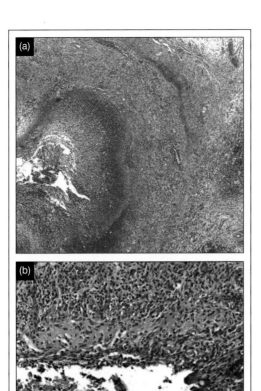

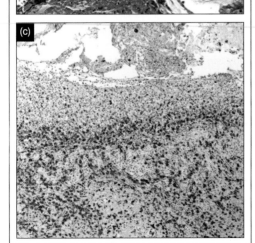

Figure 28. (**a**) Large bowel resection from a neonate with necrotizing enterocolitis showing full thickness necrosis of the bowel wall. (**b**) Higher power view to show extensive mucosal ulceration and associated acute inflammation. (**c**) Immunohistochemical staining for macrophages to show large numbers of these cells within the necrotic bowel wall. CD68 (PGM-1) immunochemistry.

Hematoxylin and eosin stains.
(**a**) Magnification ×50.
(**b**) Magnification ×200.
(**c**) Magnification ×100.

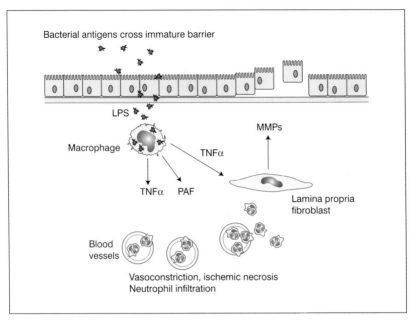

Figure 29. Putative pathogenesis of neonatal necrotizing enterocolitis. The leaky gut of a very premature baby allows bacterial components to enter the lamina propria in abundance. Some of these, such as LPS, then trigger macrophages to make TNFα and PAF. This causes vasoconstriction and ischemia, as well as increased vascular adhesion molecules, allowing neutrophils to flood into the mucosa. Cytokines also induce fibroblasts to make MMPs. The massive influx of neutrophils and locally produced MMPs then destroys the bowel wall. LPS: lipopolysaccharide; MMP: matrix metalloproteinase; PAF: platelet-activating factor; TNF: tumor necrosis factor.

Treatment

Treatment comprises cessation of enteral feeding together with both oral and intravenous antibiotic therapy. Surgical resection of the affected bowel segment might be required if it has become necrotic and/or if perforation has occurred.

Pernicious anemia

Cause

Chronic vitamin B_{12} deficiency, most commonly occurring due to autoimmune destruction of intrinsic factor-producing parietal cells within specialized gastric mucosa. Intrinsic factor is required for the absorption of vitamin B_{12} within the terminal ileum.

Age of onset	Uncommon until the fifth decade.
Gender bias	The male to female ratio is 1:1.6.
Principal clinical features	Patients usually present with unexplained macrocytic anemia or with the neurologic sequelae of vitamin B_{12} deficiency.
Epidemiology/genetics	The disease incidence is 1 in 1,000, with individuals of blood group A at higher risk.
Association with other diseases	One to three percent of patients with longstanding pernicious anemia are at significantly increased risk of developing gastric adenocarcinoma due to parietal cell loss, achlorhydria, and bacterial overgrowth, with the local production of carcinogens within the stomach. Chronic hypochlorhydria leads to secondary G-cell hyperplasia and hypergastrinemia, and can result in the development of one or more microcarcinoid tumors. There is also an increased risk of pancreatic and colonic carcinoma. Patients might develop other autoimmune diseases, such as vitiligo, Addison's disease, and autoimmune thyroid disease. Approximately 25% of patients with dermatitis herpetiformis also have autoimmune gastritis, which is not gluten responsive.
Location of lesion within bowel	Stomach
Extraintestinal manifestations	Subacute combined degeneration of the spinal cord, leading to an impaired joint position and vibration sense, together with peripheral neuropathy.
Diagnostic tests	Patients show macrocytic anemia with a low vitamin B_{12} level. Circulating parietal-cell antibodies are detectable in 90% of patients, and antibodies to intrinsic factor and to the gastrin receptor might also be present.
Major immunopathologic features	Endoscopy reveals a body-predominant or pangastritis. Histologic examination of gastric mucosal biopsies reveals chronic gastritis, with

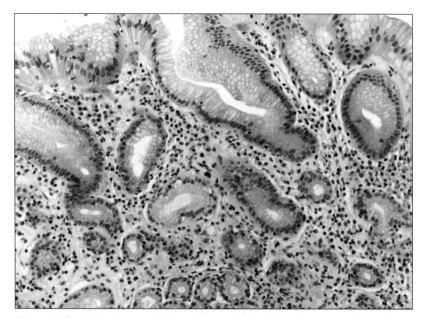

Figure 30. Gastric body mucosal biopsy from a patient with pernicious anemia, showing a mild chronic inflammatory cell infiltrate within the lamina propria, together with loss of the normal specialized body-type glands and replacement with pyloric-type mucus glands. Hematoxylin and eosin stain. Magnification ×200.

variable but often marked glandular atrophy within the specialized mucosa of the body and fundus **(Figure 30)**. This is often associated with intestinal metaplasia, and might also be associated with epithelial dysplasia and gastric adenocarcinoma.

Putative immunopathogenesis

Pernicious anemia is an autoimmune disease. Disease-specific autoantibodies target gastric parietal and zymogenic cells within the gastric glands. The autoantigens associated with this disease have been defined as those recognizing gastric H^+/K^+ ATPase and intrinsic factor.

Treatment

Vitamin B_{12} deficiency is corrected with regular vitamin B_{12} injections, and the neurologic complications may completely resolve. However, the risk of gastric adenocarcinoma remains and endoscopic follow-up might be recommended.

A difficulty is that gastric epithelial dysplasia can occur as a multifocal process, and the true extent of mucosal abnormality might therefore not be represented within random biopsies.

Post-transplant lymphoproliferative disorder

Cause	Post-transplant lymphoproliferative disorder (PTLD) is an immunosuppression-related proliferation of lymphoid cells. It shows many characteristics of lymphoma and is usually driven by Epstein–Barr virus (EBV).
Age of onset	Any
Principal clinical features	PTLD affecting the bowel can present with bowel obstruction, perforation, or intussusception.
Epidemiology/genetics	Not applicable
Association with other diseases	None, apart from the diseases that originally led to organ transplantation.
Location of lesion within bowel	Most commonly occurs within the small or large intestine. PTLD may be multifocal in nature.
Extraintestinal manifestations	Lymph nodes
Diagnostic tests	Histology (see below) and molecular clonality testing in the appropriate clinical context.
Major immunopathologic features	Histologic examination of biopsy or resection tissue reveals a high-grade proliferation of lymphoid cells, usually of B-cell phenotype and morphologically like lymphoma (**Figure 31**). The proliferation can appear polymorphous (ie, of mixed histologic appearance) or monomorphous. The former may be monoclonal or polyclonal in nature, while the latter is usually monoclonal. EBV is usually demonstrable using immunohistochemistry (eg, for latent membrane protein) or *in situ* hybridization (eg, for EBV-expressed RNA).

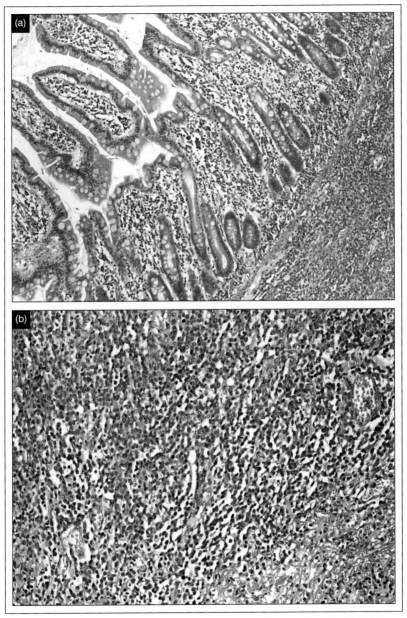

Figure 31. Small bowel showing post-transplant lymphoproliferative disorder. (a) Medium-power image showing lymphoid infiltrate within the submucosa. (b) High-power image showing the sheet-like, blast-like lymphoid infiltrate.

Hematoxylin and eosin stains. (a) Magnification ×200. (b) Magnification ×400.

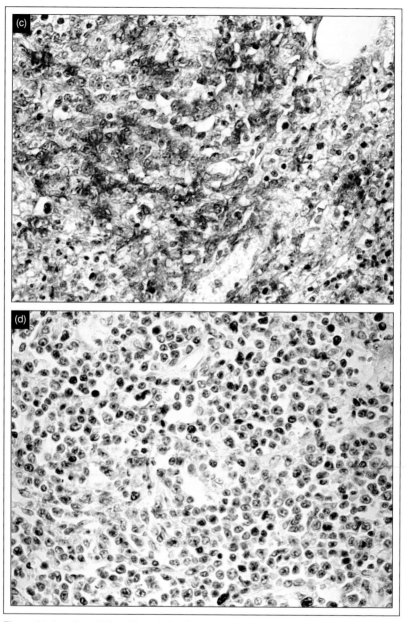

Figure 31. (continued) Small bowel showing post-transplant lymphoproliferative disorder. (**c**) Immunohistochemistry for CD20 (B-lymphocyte marker). (**d**) Immunohistochemistry for Epstein–Barr virus nuclear antigen-1.

Hematoxylin and eosin stains. (**c**) Magnification ×400. (**d**) Magnification ×400.

PTLD arising after bone marrow transplantation is usually of donor origin, while that arising after solid organ transplantation is usually of host origin.

Putative immunopathogenesis	EBV infection of B cells causes them to divide. In normal individuals, the CMI response to EBV controls the infection and kills the infected B cells, although the virus persists in a latent state. In individuals receiving immunosuppression to control transplant rejection, CMI to EBV also becomes compromised because of the non-specific nature of the immunosuppression. The infection is reactivated and B cell clones start to divide. Patients who are seronegative for EBV at the time of transplantation are particularly at risk of PTLD, presumably because of an absence of memory cells and the inability to fight a primary infection acquired after transplantation.
Treatment	Surgery is often required, particularly if bowel involvement results in an acute intra-abdominal emergency, such as perforation. Reduction of immunosuppression can be associated with a reduction in size or disappearance of the lesion. However, many cases require conventional chemotherapy and are associated with a poor prognosis.

Pouchitis

Cause	Inflammation within an ileoanal pouch constructed following colectomy, principally for UC.
Age of onset	Any
Principal clinical features	Abdominal pain, increased frequency of bowel action, and rectal bleeding. Systemic symptoms include malaise and fever.
Epidemiology/genetics	Not applicable – it is an iatrogenic disease.
Association with other diseases	Pouchitis occurs more often after surgery for UC and is very rare in patients who have had

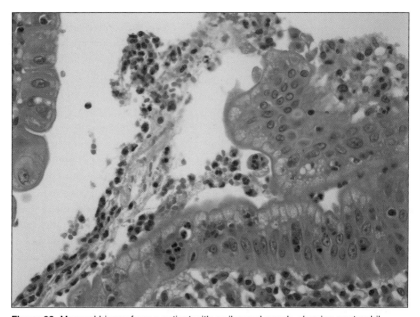

Figure 32. Mucosal biopsy from a patient with an ileoanal pouch, showing neutrophil infiltration of the surface epithelium and associated surface acute inflammatory debris. These histological features would support a clinical diagnosis of active pouchitis.
Hematoxylin and eosin stain. Magnification ×400.

a colectomy to prevent cancer, such as those with FAP.

Location of lesion within bowel

The ileum forming the pouch is the principal site of involvement, although inflammation can also develop within the ileum proximal to the pouch ("prepouch ileitis").

Extraintestinal manifestations

Extraintestinal manifestations usually associated with IBD can occur (see **Ulcerative colitis** and **Crohn's disease**, p. 142 and p. 86).

Diagnostic tests

Confident diagnosis relies upon the presence of the following triad of features:

* clinical symptoms (including systemic illness)

* endoscopically inflamed pouch mucosa

* supportive features on mucosal biopsy (**Figure 32**)

Major immunopathologic features	Acute inflammation, with neutrophils extending into the surface or crypt epithelium, and sometimes with ulceration. These changes might simulate Crohn's disease, even if the initial surgery was not performed for this condition. Villous blunting and an increase in chronic inflammatory cell numbers within the LP constitute adaptive changes and are insufficient to support a diagnosis of pouchitis. Differential diagnosis includes mucosal ischemia and mucosal prolapse.
Putative immunopathogenesis	The precise cause is unknown. The disease might develop due to changes in the function of the small intestine from absorption to storage, with secondary bacterial overgrowth. In patients who have undergone colectomy for UC, pouchitis may represent recurrent UC within the ileal mucosa that has undergone adaptive changes to a colonic phenotype. However, since the cause of UC is unknown, the cause of its possible recurrence in the adapted pouch is also unknown.
Treatment	Metronidazole can reduce or eliminate bacterial overgrowth. Probiotics have been reported to be effective. Many patients choose to have the pouch removed and replaced with an ileostomy.

Pseudomembranous colitis

Cause	Most commonly associated with broad-spectrum antibiotic therapy, leading to loss of the normal gut flora and overgrowth of toxin-producing *Clostridium difficile* bacteria.
Age of onset	Any, but a particular problem in the elderly.
Principal clinical features	Profuse diarrhea is the main symptom. Severe cases can result in a fulminant colitis.
Epidemiology/genetics	Pseudomembranous colitis may occur in a sporadic manner. Localized outbreaks can occur in hospital due to a combination of transfer of *C. difficile*

between patients and a high prevalence of broad-spectrum antibiotic usage. Pseudomembranous colitis can also cause epidemic diarrhea in daycare centers. *C. difficile* is present in 70% of infants, 3% of infants older than 1 year of age, and 2% of healthy adults.

Association with other diseases	None
Location of lesion within bowel	The condition most commonly affects the colon, although it can also affect the small bowel (pseudomembranous enterocolitis).
Extraintestinal manifestations	None
Diagnostic tests	There are a number of tests that aid diagnosis. The best is detection of *C. difficile* cytotoxin B in stools by the ability of the stool filtrate to damage fibroblasts in culture. ELISAs for the toxin in stools are also available. Stool leukocytes can be helpful, and sigmoidoscopy might reveal the characteristic yellow–white raised plaques scattered over the mucosal surface. Plain abdominal radiography might show dilated loops of bowel, and pneumatosis might be present in fulminant *C. difficile* colitis.
Major immunopathologic features	Three types of histology can be seen.

• In type 1, there is focal epithelial necrosis and exudation of fibrin and neutrophils into the lumen.

• In type 2, there are dome-shaped plaques of fibrin and cells ("volcano lesions") with normal intervening mucosa (**Figure 33**).

• In type 3, there is complete necrosis of the mucosa.

Putative immunopathogenesis	This is not directly an immune-mediated disease. Instead, the disease can be explained by the action of the two *C. difficile* toxins: toxin A is a potent

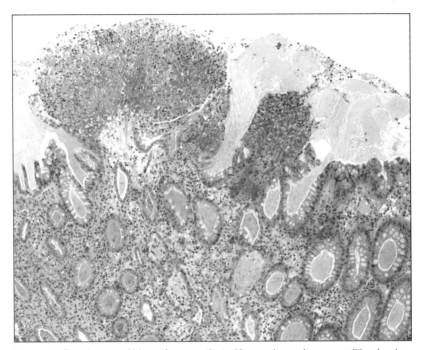

Figure 33. Rectal mucosal biopsy from a patient with pseudomembranous colitis, showing edema within the lamina propria and a characteristic "volcano lesion" comprising acute inflammatory debris issuing from the mucosal surface.
Hematoxylin and eosin stain. Magnification ×100.

enterotoxin, causing fluid secretion and epithelial necrosis; toxin B is highly cytopathic for mammalian cells. However, the interaction of toxin A with epithelial cells results in the rapid production of chemokines, which might cause neutrophils to move into the mucosa.

Treatment

Antibiotic therapy with oral vancomycin or metronidazole is usually effective, although the condition becomes recurrent in a minority of patients. Probiotics may be of some prophylactic benefit. Colectomy is rarely required if fulminant colitis supervenes.

Reflux esophagitis

Cause	Reflux of gastric acid and/or bile into the lower esophagus.
Age of onset	Any
Principal clinical features	The most common symptoms are heartburn and acid regurgitation. Esophageal strictures can also develop and cause dysphagia.
Epidemiology/genetics	Common. No known genetic predisposition.
Association with other diseases	Reflux esophagitis is commonly associated with the presence of a hiatus hernia.
Location of lesion within bowel	Lower esophagus
Extraintestinal manifestations	None
Diagnostic tests	Endoscopy reveals mucosal inflammation or ulceration and might show features in keeping with Barrett's esophagus. Monitoring of the esophageal pH is also useful.
Major immunopathologic features	Mucosal biopsy can confirm the presence of inflammation and ulceration. Mild reflux disease is particularly characterized by the presence of lymphocytes and eosinophils within the esophageal epithelium, which is a common finding in children with gastroesophageal reflux (**Figure 34**). In more severe reflux esophagitis, there can be ulceration and acute inflammation. Reflux esophagitis is a major risk factor for the development of Barrett's esophagus, which is a specialized metaplastic epithelium lining the lower esophagus, often containing goblet cells. Endoscopic surveillance of Barrett's esophagus is recommended because it is associated with a 30- to 125-fold increase in the chance of development of esophageal adenocarcinoma.
Putative immunopathogenesis	Non-specific injury to the esophagus due to acid and bile. It was thought that since *Helicobacter*

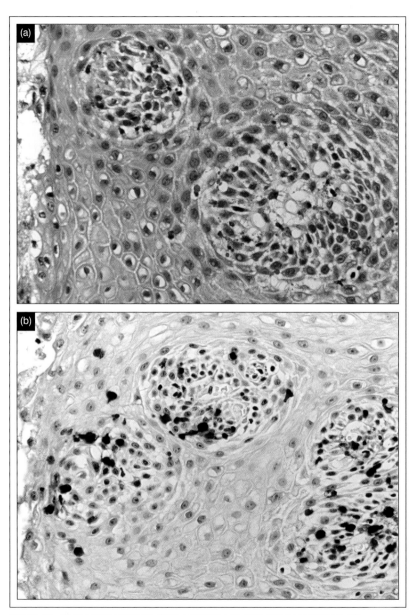

Figure 34. (**a**) Esophageal biopsy from a patient with mild gastroesophageal reflux disease, showing mild intraepithelial edema and small numbers of lymphocytes and eosinophils within the epithelium. (**b**) Immunohistochemical staining for eosinophils to highlight these cells within the esophageal epithelium.

(**a**) Hematoxylin and eosin stain. Magnification ×400. (**b**) EG2 immunohistochemistry. Magnification ×400.

pylori results in suppression of acid secretion, elimination of *H. pylori* might result in an increase in gastroesophageal reflux disease. However, there is increasing evidence that this is not the case.

Treatment	Gastric acid suppression therapy with proton-pump inhibitors is usually very effective. By maintaining the gastric pH above 4, the damaging effects of acid on the esophageal epithelium are reduced.

Refractory sprue

Cause	Unknown
Age of onset	Middle-aged and elderly individuals, although it can present in patients in their twenties.
Principal clinical features	Patients present with the same symptoms as celiac disease (see p. 68), and many have a history of celiac disease.
Epidemiology/genetics	Rare. Given the association with celiac disease, most patients are HLA-DQ2 positive.
Association with other diseases	Refractory sprue is probably a cryptic T-cell lymphoma, presenting clinically between celiac disease and overt EATL (see p. 96). It is associated with uncommon manifestations of celiac disease, such as ulcerative jejunitis and mesenteric lymph-node cavitation.
Location of lesion within bowel	Duodenum and upper jejunum
Extraintestinal manifestations	Many patients become severely malnourished.
Diagnostic tests	Although there might be some initial clinical improvement on a gluten-free diet, refractory sprue does not respond significantly to a strict gluten-free diet. Around 80% of patients are antiendomysial antibody positive. Analysis of TCR rearrangement in biopsies reveals a clonal pattern,

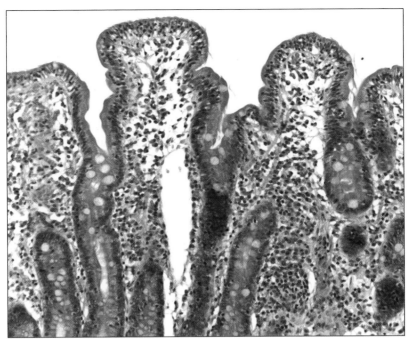

Figure 35. Duodenal mucosal biopsy from a patient with refractory sprue, showing partial villous blunting, crypt hyperplasia, and an increase in intraepithelial lymphocyte numbers. The appearances are essentially consistent with those of active celiac disease.
Hematoxylin and eosin stain. Magnification ×200.

showing the malignant nature of the condition. Immunohistochemistry on frozen sections shows a very unusual population of IELs that are surface CD3, CD4, and CD8 negative, but contain cytoplasmic CD3.

Major immunopathologic features

Duodenal or jejunal biopsy can reveal mucosal remodeling with loss of villi and crypt hyperplasia to give the classic "flat mucosa". There is an increase in chronic inflammatory cell numbers in the LP and an increase in the density of IELs (**Figure 35**).

Putative Immunopathogenesis

By analogy with celiac disease, the lesion is probably driven by activated T cells. Whereas in celiac disease these are CD4+ LP T cells responding to gluten peptides, this is not the case in refractory sprue, since there is little improvement on a gluten-free diet. The role that the neoplastic IELs play in the lesion is not understood, since there have been few functional studies on these cells.

Treatment

Refractory sprue is a serious condition. Some patients respond to steroids and other immunosuppressives such as methotrexate or azathioprine, but many become severely malnourished, require parenteral nutrition, and die.

Selective immunoglobulin A deficiency

Cause

The failure to produce IgA, the major Ig class secreted at mucosal surfaces, especially the gastrointestinal tract.

Age of onset

IgA deficiency is a primary immunodeficiency and so is present from birth.

Principal clinical features

Most patients are completely well because of compensatory elevated mucosal IgM responses – as polymeric IgM contains J chain, it is able to bind to the polymeric Ig receptor on the baso-lateral aspect of epithelial cells and be transported into the gut lumen. However, some patients are susceptible to high rates of infection of bacterial pathogens in the gut, airways, and urogenital tract. *Giardia lamblia* infections, nodular lymphoid hyperplasia, non-specific enteropathy, and bacterial overgrowth are seen in the gut of IgA-deficient patients, which can produce steatorrhea and diarrhea.

Epidemiology/genetics

Incidence of around 1 in 333 within white populations. IgA deficiency occurs in families, suggesting autosomal inheritance.

Association with other diseases

Selective IgA deficiency can be associated with several other diseases, mainly autoimmune diseases such as pernicious anemia, Addison's disease, autoimmune thyroid disease, systemic lupus erythematosus, rheumatoid arthritis, primary biliary cirrhosis, autoimmune hepatitis, and celiac disease. Patients with IgA deficiency and a clinical history suggestive of celiac disease will not have serum IgA antigliadin and antiendomysial/tTG antibodies, and so might give false-negative serology results.

Location of lesion within bowel	Small bowel
Extraintestinal manifestations	The generalized lack of IgA can lead to recurrent infections in the airways and urogenital tract.
Diagnostic tests	The serum IgA level is either zero or almost zero (<0.05 g/L).
Major immunopathologic features	Small-bowel biopsy might show an essentially normal morphologic appearance (including the presence of IgM plasma cells within the LP) or a variable degree of villous blunting and, occasionally, a flat mucosa.
Putative immunopathogenesis	It is assumed that IgA deficiency, with insufficient compensatory IgM, leads to defective secretory immunity in some patients. IgA is important in immunity to *G. lamblia* since, by agglutinating the organism, it prevents it attaching to the surface epithelium. It is not clear whether IgA in the gut plays any role in keeping the small bowel clear of colonic flora, so bacterial overgrowth remains unexplained.
Treatment	Treatment might not be required, but supportive therapy (eg, treatment of infections) might be needed.

Severe combined immunodeficiency disease

Cause	This is a heterogeneous group of disorders characterized by a block in T-cell differentiation, which is variably associated with defective

development of B cells and natural killer cells. The majority of severe combined immunodeficiency disease (SCID) patients have no T cells, but deficiencies in MHC class II molecules or the TCR signaling molecule ZAP70 can lead to a SCID phenotype with normal numbers of T cells.

Age of onset

Usually within the first few weeks of life.

Principal clinical features

Lymphopenia, hypogammaglobulinemia, recurrent severe infections, and failure to thrive. Gastrointestinal tract involvement leads to diarrhea, malabsorption, and infection with many different organisms (bacteria, viruses, fungi, and protozoa). Other gastrointestinal tract features include esophageal atresia and imperforate anus.

Epidemiology/genetics

The incidence is about 1 in 75,000–100,000 live births. The condition can be inherited in either an autosomal-recessive or X-linked manner. Mutations in the enzyme adenosine deaminase, common cytokine receptor γ chain, IL-7 receptor α chain, *RAG1* or *RAG2* genes (the genes that reorganize T-cell and B-cell DNA to make T- and B-cell receptors), and CD45 (common leukocyte antigen) all result in a SCID phenotype.

Association with other diseases

SCID is not associated with other diseases, but other mixed immunodeficiency states may be present, eg, Wiskott–Aldrich syndrome (associated with eczema and thrombocytopenia) and ataxia telangiectasia (associated with lymphoreticular malignancy).

Location of lesion within bowel

Small and large intestine

Extraintestinal manifestations

As well as severe diarrhea, affected children suffer from oral candidiasis, interstitial pneumonitis, and infections from *Pneumocystis carinii* and *Aspergillus*, *Listeria*, and *Legionella* species, as well as herpes viruses.

Diagnostic tests

The diagnosis can be established using tests for Ig levels and blood T-cell numbers and function.

Major immunopathologic features	Endoscopic examination reveals friable intestinal mucosa. Histologic examination of mucosal biopsies reveals partial villous atrophy (small intestine) and periodic acid-Schiff (PAS)-positive macrophages, but no lymphocytes or plasma cells within the LP.
Putative immunopathogenesis	SCID patients show that T cells are necessary for survival. In their absence, patients suffer from overwhelming systemic and mucosal infections that almost invariably lead to death by 1 year of age.
Treatment	Supportive therapy (eg, treatment of infections and Ig treatment) is useful. Bone marrow transplantation provides the only hope of a long-term cure. SCID patients without an HLA-identical donor can be treated with a haploidentical donor as long as T cells are removed from the inoculum to prevent GVHD (see p. 103). In the absence of GVHD, about 75% of patients survive.

Trichuriasis

Cause	The parasitic nematode *Trichuris trichiura* (whipworm).
Age of onset	Any, but more common in children.
Principal clinical features	Most patients are asymptomatic, but common symptoms in heavy infection include anemia, chronic dysentery with blood and mucus, and rectal prolapse.
Epidemiology/genetics	The organism has a worldwide distribution, but is more common in the tropics. Infection occurs via the fecal–oral route. In endemic areas, worm burden in children is highly skewed, with 5% of patients having 95% of the parasites. The reason for this is unknown. In the developed world, it may be more common in individuals living in institutions because of developmental difficulties, or in immigrants from the developing world.

Association with other diseases	None
Location of lesion within bowel	The worm lives in the colon.
Extraintestinal manifestations	None
Diagnostic tests	Diagnosis relies on the identification of eggs of the parasite in stools.
Major immunopathologic features	Colonoscopic biopsies reveal an essentially normal colonic mucosa, with long, mucus-filled glands. Worms may be seen with their heads buried in the epithelium.
Putative immunopathogenesis	Although it is widely considered that parasites damage the gut, there is remarkably little damage to the colon in patients with trichuriasis, even in children with heavy infections. Mechanical injury to the epithelium by the invading nematode undoubtedly leads to blood loss and a break in the epithelial barrier. The mucosa is also filled with IgE-positive mast cells, and there is evidence for an ongoing local IgE-mediated type I hypersensitivity response. Release of mast-cell mediators will cause fluid secretion, very much as in allergic proctitis (see p. 52).
Treatment	Mebendazole or pyrantel-oxantel are effective therapies.

Tropical sprue

Cause	The precise cause is unclear, but it is likely to be infection of the small bowel with one of several different organisms (possibly toxin-producing), together with nutritional deficiency.
Age of onset	Any

Principal clinical features	Diarrhea, abdominal bloating, and nutritional deficiency. The disease can be chronic, with relapses and remissions, and might not spontaneously improve among affected travelers returning to non-tropical areas.
Epidemiology/genetics	In the developing world, the majority of healthy individuals show inflammatory changes and some villus atrophy in their upper bowel. It is unclear whether tropical sprue is part of this spectrum or a different condition.
Association with other diseases	None
Location of lesion within bowel	Jejunum, and can extend to involve the ileum.
Extraintestinal manifestations	None
Diagnostic tests	There is no diagnostic test to discriminate tropical sprue from any other disease of the upper gastrointestinal tract.
Major immunopathologic features	Small-bowel biopsy reveals features very similar to celiac disease, with mucosal remodeling and an increase in both IELs and chronic inflammatory cells within the LP. Tropical sprue is gluten unresponsive.
Putative immunopathogenesis	By analogy with celiac disease (see p. 68), the mucosal changes can be driven by a mucosal Th1 response to low-grade enteric infections.
Treatment	Antibiotic therapy (eg, tetracycline) is usually required, together with nutritional supplements (especially folic acid and vitamin B_{12}). Further supportive care (eg, rehydration) might be needed in severe cases.

Ulcerative colitis

Cause	Unknown
Age of onset	Any. The peak age of onset is in young adults, with a second smaller peak in the sixth and seventh decades.
Principal clinical features	Abdominal pain and diarrhea, often associated with blood or mucus.
Epidemiology/genetics	Like Crohn's disease, UC has a familial risk. Associations with certain MHC class II alleles have been shown in different populations, but the association varies with the group studied. The incidence is around 1 in 500–1,000 and, unlike Crohn's disease, UC has a worldwide distribution. A prior history of smoking is protective, as is prior appendicectomy. It also appears that appendicectomy after the development of proctitis results in much less severe disease and less colectomies.
Association with other diseases	Colonic glandular epithelial dysplasia and colorectal adenocarcinoma can occur, with the highest risk being in patients with longstanding UC (especially with disease duration >10 years) and in cases of total colonic involvement. Severe UC can lead to toxic megacolon and perforation, which can be life-threatening.
Location of lesion within bowel	The disease most commonly affects the rectum and a variable proportion of the colon, usually with a continuous distribution. Occasionally, proctitis is associated with cecal inflammation (cecal "patch lesion"), with normal intervening colon. The terminal ileum can also become inflamed ("backwash ileitis").
Extraintestinal manifestations	Several other organs can be involved, in a similar way to Crohn's disease. These include the liver (sclerosing cholangitis; said to be more common in association with UC than Crohn's disease), eye (uveitis, episcleritis), skin (erythema

nodosum, pyoderma gangrenosum), and joints (seronegative arthropathy).

Diagnostic tests

Diagnosis is made with a combination of clinical history and the endoscopic features of proctitis or colitis. Patients with UC have raised levels of antibodies to neutrophil cytoplasmic proteins, whereas those with Crohn's disease have raised levels of ASCA. By carrying out both tests, guidance for diagnosis can be made, but a definitive diagnosis still requires histology, clinical history, and disease course. During exacerbations of disease, serum albumin is low and the erythrocyte sedimentation rate and levels of CRP are raised.

Major immunopathologic features

UC shows a characteristic histologic appearance of acute and chronic inflammation, with cryptitis and crypt abscesses, together with features indicating chronicity (eg, glandular architectural distortion) (**Figure 36**). Except in severe cases, lesions are restricted to the mucosa.

Putative Immunopathogenesis

UC has many of the features of an antibody-mediated, organ-specific autoimmune disease. The diseased mucosa is densely infiltrated with IgG plasma cells, and deposition of IgG1 and complement can be visualized on colonic epithelium. The pathological appearance of UC is almost exactly mirrored by rabbit immune complex colitis, where disease is induced by a massive Arthus reaction in the colonic wall. There has, however, been a lack of progress in defining putative autoantigens in UC. Increased cytokines in the mucosa (as a result of the neutrophil and macrophage infiltrate) up-regulate the expression of adhesion molecules on vascular endothelium so that more inflammatory cells are recruited from the blood. Cytokines also activate resident fibroblasts to secrete matrix-degrading enzymes (MMPs), which are probably responsible for ulceration. Inflammation results in the destruction of the epithelial barrier, with ingress of luminal contents

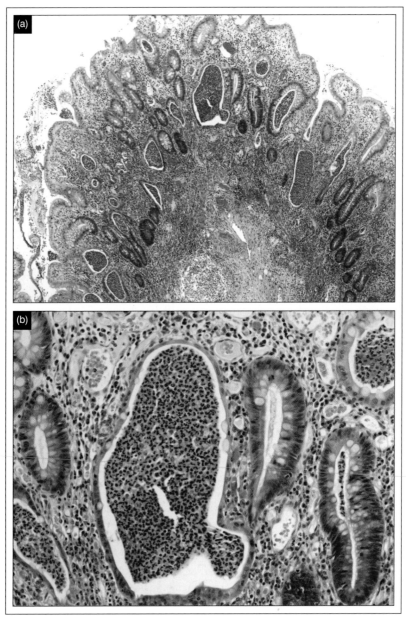

Figure 36. (a) Large-bowel mucosa and submucosa from colectomy for severe ulcerative colitis, showing acute and chronic inflammation within the lamina propria, with crypt abscess formation. (b) Higher-power view to show several crypt abscesses.

Hematoxylin and eosin stains. (a) Magnification ×50. (b) Magnification ×200.

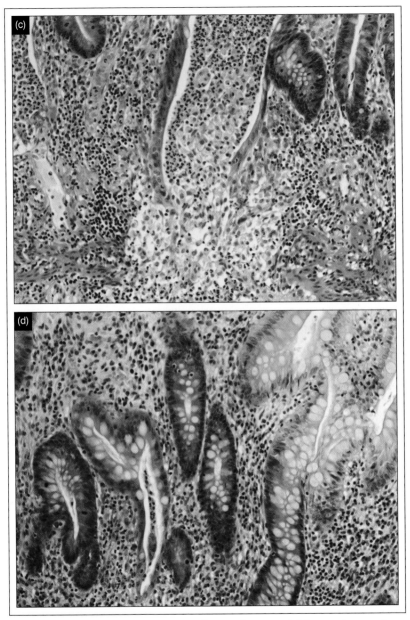

Figure 36 (continued). (**c,d**) Higher-power views to show a cryptolytic granuloma and glandular distortion, respectively.

Hematoxylin and eosin stains. (**c,d**) Magnification ×200.

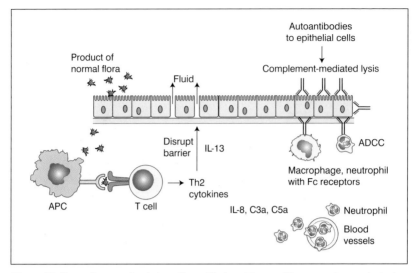

Figure 37. The pathogenesis of ulcerative colitis is not known. There may be an atypical Th2 response and IL-13 can disrupt the barrier. Antibodies directed against epithelial cells have also been well-documented and could destroy epithelial cells via complement or ADCC. Complement activation will also cause neutrophils to move into the mucosa. ADCC: antibody-dependent cellular cytotoxicity; APC: antigen-presenting cell; IL: interleukin; Th: T-helper cell.

into the mucosa and subsequent non-specific injury (**Figure 37**). Recent studies also suggest that T-cell-driven injury might also play a role, with an atypical Th2 response occurring in the mucosa and increased production of IL-13. IL-13 can cause the gut epithelium to become leaky.

Treatment

The disease is cured by colectomy. However, anti-inflammatory therapy with sulfasalazines and/or steroids is the mainstay of medical treatment. Patients with proven dysplasia or carcinoma, or those at high risk for development of these complications, usually require total colectomy. Total colectomy might also be required in patients with severe colitis that is unresponsive to medical therapy, particularly if toxic megacolon supervenes. Cyclosporin A is highly effective in patients with severe disease.

Vasculitis

Cause	Vasculitis is caused by immune-mediated damage to blood vessel walls, often with associated luminal thrombosis.
Age of onset	Any
Principal clinical features	Vasculitis in the gut can cause abdominal pain and malabsorption, with severe cases presenting with localized or widespread bowel ischemia or infarction. Vasculitis involving the gastrointestinal tract is often part of a systemic vasculitic process, often with multiple organ involvement and associated clinical features (eg, skin rash, renal failure).
Epidemiology/genetics	Not applicable
Association with other diseases	Many different diseases can cause vasculitis, including idiopathic Henoch–Schönlein syndrome, polyarteritis nodosum, Kawasaki disease, Wegener's granulomatosis, Churg–Strauss vasculitis, Behçet's disease, and autoimmune diseases such as systemic lupus erythematosus and Sjögren's syndrome. Small- and medium-sized vessels are subject to attack and so there is involvement of many different organs throughout the body.
Location of lesion within bowel	Any part of the gut.
Extraintestinal manifestations	Common. Distribution depends upon the underlying nature of the vasculitic process (see above).
Diagnostic tests	Accurate diagnosis relies upon clear clinical evidence of one or more characteristically involved sites. The erythrocyte sedimentation rate and levels of serum CRP are raised.
Major immunopathologic features	Mucosal biopsy might show ischemic changes (**Figure 38**), but the primary vasculitic lesion (eg, a leukocytoclastic or granulomatous vasculitis) might not be identified unless submucosa is included in

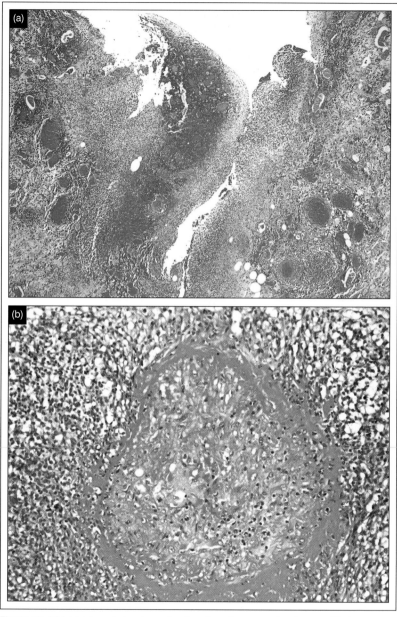

Figure 38. (**a**) Large bowel showing extensive ulceration secondary to vasculitis in polyarteritis nodosa. (**b**) Small artery showing fibrinoid necrosis of its wall and reactive intimal proliferation.

Hematoxylin and eosin stains. (**a**) Magnification ×100. (**b**) Magnification ×400.

the specimen. Definitive diagnosis is usually more straightforward within resection specimens.

Putative immunopathogenesis	Vasculitis is usually an autoimmune disease. It can be due to immune complexes being deposited in vessels, or to production of autoantibodies to vessel antigens.
Treatment	Anti-inflammatory therapy (eg, with steroids, cyclophosphamide, or azathioprine) can produce dramatic results. However, a fulminant presentation or serious multisystem involvement might still be associated with a poor outcome unless diagnosis and initiation of treatment are prompt.

Whipple's disease

Cause	The bacterium *Tropheryma whipplei*.
Age of onset	Most commonly within the fourth and fifth decades of life.
Gender bias	Males are more commonly affected than females.
Principal clinical features	This is a multisystem disorder, with the main clinical features being fever, polymyalgia, malabsorption, and lymphadenopathy. Hepatosplenomegaly, pericarditis, pleural or pulmonary infection, and cardiac valve vegetations can also occur.
Epidemiology/genetics	The disease is most common within North America and Europe, but is still a very rare condition. *T. whipplei* DNA can be isolated from saliva, gastric juice, and duodenal biopsies of healthy individuals, suggesting that exposure may be common.
Association with other diseases	None
Location of lesion within bowel	When the bowel is involved, the jejunum and ileum are the most commonly affected sites.

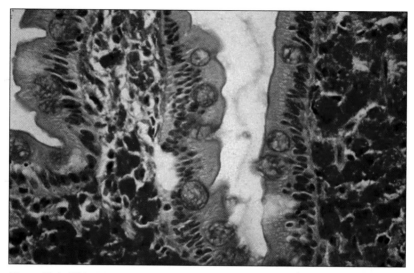

Figure 39. In Whipple's disease, the lamina propria is filled with macrophages containing the Whipple's bacteria, which stain red with periodic acid-Schiff.
Magnification ×400.

Extraintestinal manifestations	See above
Diagnostic tests	Histology was once the classic way to diagnose infections. However, the organism was finally cultured in 2000, so antibodies are now available for immunohistochemical detection of the organism in tissues. Polymerase chain reaction-based technologies are also being used for diagnosis.
Major immunopathologic features	Biopsy of involved tissues reveals PAS-positive material within macrophages, eg, within the LP of the intestinal mucosa (**Figure 39**). Electron microscopy reveals that the PAS-positive material is collections of phagocytosed bacteria. Within the small intestine, villous blunting can be seen and collections of lipid might also be present, possibly secondary to lymphatic channel blockage. Granulomas may be present within involved lymph nodes and other organs.

Putative immunopathogenesis	There appears to be some defect in Th1 immunity, which allows the bacterium to survive in the tissues. In the absence of effective immunity, the organism multiplies within macrophages in the bowel wall.
Treatment	Antibiotic therapy with trimethoprim-sulfamethoxazole usually leads to a dramatic clinical response.

Yersinia enterocolitis

Cause	The cause is intestinal infection with the Gram-negative bacilli *Yersinia enterocolitica* or *Y. paratuberculosis*.
Age of onset	Any
Principal clinical features	The clinical presentation is varied, but most commonly includes abdominal pain, diarrhea, and pyrexia, associated with enteritis and/or colitis. Mesenteric adenitis can simulate acute appendicitis, and several outbreaks have led to clusters of appendicectomies.
Epidemiology/genetics	The disease occurs more commonly in cold climates. Yersiniae exist as a reservoir in wild animals and, unusually, can grow at low temperatures. Transmission of the organisms usually occurs via contaminated food or drinking water.
Association with other diseases	None
Location of lesion within bowel	The entire small and large intestine can be involved or the disease might be limited, eg, to the terminal ileum and cecum.
Extraintestinal manifestations	Arthritis and erythema nodosum may occur.

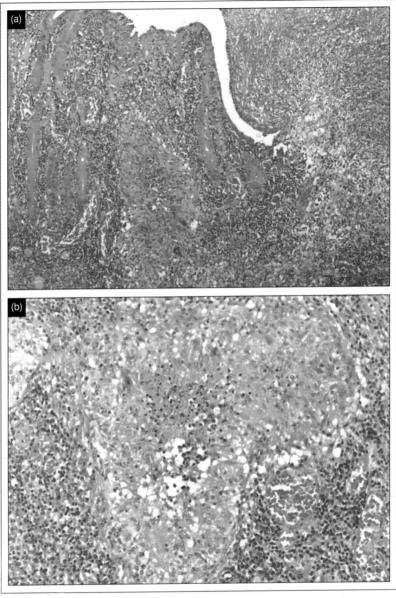

Figure 40. (a) Terminal ileum from a right hemicolectomy specimen removed due to *Yersinia* enterocolitis. Marked transmural acute and chronic inflammation is present (mucosa and submucosa shown here), with ulceration. (b) Higher-power view to show a granuloma within the inflamed bowel wall.

Hematoxylin and eosin stains. (a) Magnification ×100. (b) Magnification ×200.

| Diagnostic tests | Isolation of the organisms from stools is definitive. Serological tests for anti-*Yersinia* antibodies are also useful. |

Major immunopathologic features — Macroscopic examination of resected bowel shows features mimicking Crohn's disease. Microscopic examination of resection specimens classically reveals marked lymphoid hyperplasia, often with microabscesses contained within the lymphoid follicles. Granulomatous inflammation might be present, causing further potential confusion with Crohn's disease. Mucosal biopsies reveal the features of a non-specific colitis (**Figure 40**).

Putative immunopathogenesis — Yersiniae take advantage of the gut's immune system to invade the body. M cells overlying the PPs phagocytose particles and antigens from the gut lumen and transport them into the subepithelial dome, where there are abundant APCs and T and B cells. Yersiniae target M cells and so are transported into the PP. In the PP, they target macrophages using a specific bacterial surface protein, which binds to an integrin on macrophages. After a bacterium is ingested it secretes a number of proteins that prevent the macrophage from killing the bacterium, which can then multiply intracellularly. Persistence of bacteria, however, also elicits a vigorous Th1 response to the organisms, which produces the Crohn's-like pathology in the gut wall.

Treatment — Infection can require bowel resection, but may also be self limiting. Antibiotic treatment (eg, tetracycline) might be required in severe cases.

Glossary

A

Accessory molecule

A molecule that links **T cells** and **antigen-presenting cells (APCs)** following **T-cell receptor (TCR)** binding. Examples include **CD4, CD8, CD28**, and **lymphocyte function-associated antigen (LFA)1**.

Adjuvant

A substance that, when mixed with an **antigen**, makes the antigen more immunogenic (ie, causes it to elicit a larger immune response). In humans, particles of aluminum hydroxide (alum) are used as adjuvants. Dead vaccines, such as diphtheria–pertussis–tetanus (DPT) are given with alum.

Afferent lymphatics

The network of vessels that take **lymph** from the skin and gut to the lymph nodes.

Affinity

The ability of a **T-cell receptor (TCR)** or an **antibody** molecule to bind to its given peptide/**major histocompatibility complex (MHC)** molecule or **antigen**. High-affinity receptors bind strongly, while low-affinity receptors bind weakly.

Allogeneic

An allogeneic transplant is one that is made between two unrelated individuals.

Anergy

When **T** and **B cells** with specificity for **antigens** are still present in the body, but are not functional.

Antibody

Molecules made by **plasma cells** that mediate **humoral immunity**.

Antibody-dependent cellular cytotoxicity

A type of cell killing. Cells such as **macrophages** have Fc receptors, which they use to bind **antibodies** through the **constant (C) region**. If the antibody is bound to another cell through its **variable (V) region** then the antibody links the macrophage to the antibody-coated cell, and signaling through the Fc receptor triggers the macrophage to produce molecules that kill the antibody-coated cell.

Antigen	A molecule that generates an immune response. This can be through an infection or an organ transplant. In autoimmune disease, self proteins become antigens.
Antigen-presenting cell (APC)	Any cell that can present an **antigen** to a **T cell**. B cells, **dendritic cells**, and **macrophages** are all APCs.
Apoptosis	Programmed cell death; the capacity of any cell to kill itself in response to changing signals in the microenvironment.
Apthous	A term used to describe the small **ulcers** with punched-out centers that are found in the **mucosa** in early Crohn's disease. Oral apthous ulcers are also a feature of celiac disease.
Arthropathy	Inflammation of the joints.
Arthus reaction	A type III **hypersensitivity** reaction where immune complexes form in the skin, fix **complement**, and induce **neutrophil** infiltration into the tissues.
Ascites	The fluid that accumulates in the peritoneal cavity when blood flow through the liver is obstructed.
Atherosclerosis	The formation of fatty plaques in the blood vessels.
Atopy	The allergic state in which individuals are predisposed to **type I hypersensitivity** (eg, asthma, **eczema**, hay fever).
Autoimmunity	Inflammatory destruction of one or several of an individual's cells or tissues caused by their own immune system.

B

B cell	A **lymphocyte** that comes from the bone marrow and which is important in **antibody**-mediated immunity.
Barrett's esophagus	A change in the lining tissue of the lower esophagus from squamous to glandular type. A premalignant condition predisposing to esophageal adenocarcinoma.

C

Cachexia

Weight loss and wasting.

Capsule

The area of fibrous tissue around a **lymph node** or the **spleen**.

CARD15

See **NOD2.**

CD

See **cluster of differentiation.**

CD28

An accessory molecule on the surface of **T cells** that binds to **CD80** on **antigen-presenting cells (APCs).**

CD3

A complex of proteins that are important in transmitting a signal to the nucleus to initiate **T-cell** activation. CD3 is only found on the surface of **T cells.**

CD4 T cells

Those **T cells** that are important in cell-mediated immunity (CMI) and secrete **cytokines**, and which help **B cells** make **antibodies.**

CD8 T cells

Those **T cells** that can kill tumor cells and virally infected cells. Often known as cytotoxic T cells.

CD80/CD86

Co-stimulatory accessory molecules on **antigen-presenting cells (APCs)** that bind to receptors **(CD28, cytotoxic T-lymphocyte antigen [CTLA]4)** on **T cells** and which control the extent of the T cell response.

Chemokine

A molecule made by a cell that induces the migration of any other cell in a directional fashion (chemotaxis).

Cholestasis

Failure of bile to drain via the bile ducts either within or outside the liver.

Class I major histocompatibility complex (MHC) molecules

Products of the **MHC** on the surface of **antigen-presenting cells (APCs)** major histocompatibility complex that can bind small peptides for presentation to **CD8 T cells.**

Class II major histocompatibility complex (MHC) molecules

Products of the **MHC** on the surface of **antigen-presenting cells (APCs)** major histocompatibility complex that can bind small peptides for presentation to **CD4 T cells.**

Clonal	Derived from a single cell.
Clonal deletion	*See* **negative selection**.
Clonal expansion	The crucial part of the immune response, when individual clones of **T cells** or **B cells** responding to **antigens** undergo massive proliferation early in the immune response.
Cluster of differentiation (CD)	A nomenclature used to designate surface molecules and the **antibodies** that recognize these surface molecules.
Complement	A complex family of molecules that bind to **antibodies** when they themselves bind their **antigen**. The end stage of complement activation is a complex of proteins that punch holes in the surface of the cell to which the antibody is bound. Complement components that are released during the activation cascade, such as C3a and C5a, are highly chemotactic for **neutrophils**.
Constant (C) region	The part of **heavy chains** and **light chains** of antibody molecules that do not vary between individuals.
Cortex	The outer region of the **thymus** or a **lymph node**.
Crypts of Lieberkuhn	The **glands** in the small intestine full of proliferating **epithelial** cells that migrate from the crypts onto the surface of the **villus**.
Cytokine antigen (CTLA)4	A soluble molecule made by a cell, which binds to receptors on adjacent cells and changes their function.
Cytotoxic T-lymphocyte	An accessory molecule on **T cells** that binds to **CD86** on **antigen-presenting cells** (**APCs**) and whose function is to inhibit T cell activation.

D

Defensins	A family of highly cationic small peptides made by neutrophils and by **Paneth cells** in the gut. Defensins can kill pathogenic bacteria.
Delayed-type hypersensitivity	*See* **type IV hypersensitivity**.

Dendritic cell	A cell derived from the bone marrow that can present fragments of **antigens** to **T cells**.
Dyspepsia	Heartburn.
Dysphagia	Difficulty in swallowing.

E

Eczema	Inflammation of the skin, which may become "crusty" in chronic cases.
Edema	Excess fluid within the interstitial tissues.
Enteropathy	Inflammation of the small or large intestine.
Eosinophil	Blood-borne specialized polymorphs that are associated with type I, **IgE**-mediated **hypersensitivity**.
Eosinophilia	An abundance of **eosinophils** in the blood or tissues.
Eotaxin	A **chemokine** made by many cell types, which attracts **eosinophils** into tissues.
Episcleritis	Inflammation of the sclera, resulting in a red and painful eye that is sensitive to light.
Epithelium	The single layer of cells that lines the surface of the gut. It contains two main cell types, absorptive epithelial cells (enterocytes) and **goblet cells**. Goblet cells secrete the mucus that lines the surface of the epithelium.
Erythema nodosum	Lumpy swelling of the skin, especially occurring on the shins.
E-selectin	An adhesion molecule, the expression of which is increased on the lining of blood vessels at sites of inflammation. It recognizes sugar residues on molecules on the surface of white blood cells so that white cells in the blood stick to blood vessels and migrate through the vessel wall into the tissue.

F

F(ab')2

The part of the **antibody** molecule at the N terminus, made up of **heavy chains** and **light chains**, which binds **antigen**.

Fc

The part of the **heavy chain** of an **antibody** molecule at the carboxy terminus that does not bind **antigen**. Many types of cells have Fc receptors.

Fibrosis

Deposition of excess extracellular matrix (mainly collagen and elastin) within tissues, leading to scar formation.

Fistula

An abnormal communication between two **epithelial**-lined surfaces. This may occur between bowel loops or between the bowel and the skin or bladder.

Follicle

An area of organized lymphoid tissue with a **T-cell** and a **B-cell** zone.

Follicle-associated epithelium (FAE)

The specialized **epithelium** that overlies **Peyer's patches (PPs)** in the intestine.

Follicular dendritic cell

A specialized type of **cell** found in **germinal centers (GCs)** which presents **antigens** to B cells.

G

Germinal center (GC)

A zone of rapidly dividing **B cells** within the **follicles** where **B cells** undergo **isotype switching** and **affinity** maturation.

Giant cell

The fusion of a number of **macrophages** into a single cell with multiple nuclei, characteristically associated with **granulomas**.

Glands

When used in association with the intestine, another term for crypts.

Goblet cell

The **epithelial** cells that secrete mucus in the intestine.

Gram	A stain used to classify bacteria. Bacteria such as *Escherichia coli*, with an outer **lipopolysaccharide (LPS)** membrane in their walls, are Gram negative. Bacteria such as *Clostridia* species, with thick peptidoglycan cells walls, are Gram positive.
Granuloma	An organized accumulation of **macrophages**. Macrophages fuse and form epithelioid **giant cells**.

H

Heavy chain	Part of an **antibody** molecule that dictates the antibody class.
Heterozygote	An individual having different copies of a gene from each parent.
Hiatus hernia	The presence of part of the stomach within the chest cavity, resulting in impairment of the gastroesophageal sphincter.
High endothelial venules (HEVs)	The specialized vessels in **lymph nodes** and **Peyer's patches (PPs)** where **lymphocytes** move from the blood across the vessel wall into the lymph nodes.
Histamine	A molecule made by **mast cells** that mediates many of the features of allergies, such as itching, **edema**, vasodilation, and smooth muscle contraction.
Homozygote	An individual having identical copies of a gene from each parent.
5-Hydroxytryptamine	*See* **serotonin**.
Hyperglycemia	Abnormally high blood sugar concentration.
Hyperplasia	An increase in size, as in crypt hyperplasia of celiac disease.
Hypersensitivity	An immune response that causes tissue damage.
Hyperuricemia	An abnormally high concentration of uric acid within the blood.
Hypogammaglobulinemia	An abnormally low concentration of **immunoglobulins (Igs)** within the blood.
Hypoglycemia	Abnormally low blood sugar concentration.

I

Iatrogenic	An iatrogenic disease is one caused by a medical or surgical treatment.
Immediate hypersensitivity	*See* **type I hypersensitivity**.
Immunoglobulin (Ig)	Another word for **antibody**.
Immunoglobulin (Ig)A	The major **antibody** produced at **mucosal** surfaces.
Immunoglobulin (Ig)D	A type of antibody on the surface of newly made B cells. It has the same specificity as the IgM on the surface of the same cell, but is not secreted after B cell activation.
Immunoglobulin (Ig)E	Present in trace amounts in serum, important in allergies because it binds to **mast cells**.
Immunoglobulin (Ig)G	The major **antibody** present in serum.
Immunoglobulin (Ig)M	The first **antibody** made in an immune response and also present at **mucosal** surfaces. IgM production in the gut is high in **IgA** deficient patients, keeping the gut free from infections.
Innate immunity	The primary immune defenses of the body, such as mucus layers, **neutrophils**, stomach acid, and lysozymes. **Toll-like receptors (TLRs)** on cells are also part of the innate immune response.
α4β7 Integrin	A molecule present on the surface of T cells and B cells derived from **Peyer's patch (PP)** which controls the migration of these cells into the **lamina propria (LP)** by binding to **mucosal addressin cell adhesion molecule (MAdCAM)1** on blood vessels in the LP.
Integrin	Cell surface molecules involved in the adhesion of leukocytes to extracellular matrix and to molecules expressed on **endothelial** cells and **antigen-presenting cells (APCs)**.

Intercellular cell adhesion molecule (ICAM)1	An adhesion molecule on **antigen-presenting cells (APCs)** that binds to **lymphocyte function-associated antigen (LFA)1** on **T cells**. ICAM1 is also present on the surface of blood vessels, especially in inflamed sites. **Lymphocytes** in the blood stick to blood vessels using ICAM1 and migrate through the vessel wall into the tissue.
Interferon (IFN)γ	A **cytokine** made by **T cells** that has antiviral activity, but which also has many effects on the immune system, such as activating **macrophages** and increasing the expression of **class II major histocompatibility complex (MHC) molecules** on **antigen-presenting cells (APCs)** and **epithelial** cells.
Interleukin (IL)-1	A **cytokine** made by activated **macrophages** that is important in helping **T cells** initiate the immune response, but is much more important as a mediator of inflammation and fever. It also increases **vascular adhesion molecule** expression on **endothelial** cells.
Interleukin (IL)-2	A **cytokine** made by activated **T cells** that binds to a receptor on the same T cell and drives T cell **clonal expansion** via an autocrine growth pathway.
Interleukin (IL)-3	A **cytokine** which promotes the growth of mast cells.
Interleukin (IL)-4	A **cytokine** made by **T-helper cell type II (Th2) cells** and **mast cells** that makes **B cells** secrete **immunoglobulin (Ig)E**.
Interleukin (IL)-5	A **cytokine** made by **T-helper cell type II (Th2) cells** and **eosinophils** that is an important eosinophil growth factor and chemoattractant.
Interleukin (IL)-6	A **cytokine** made by many different types of cells in inflammation and which is the mediator that stimulates C-reactive protein (CRP) production by hepatocytes.
Interleukin (IL)-8	A **chemokine** made by many cells that is very chemotactic for **neutrophils**.

| Interleukin (IL)-10 | A **cytokine** made by **T-helper cell type II (Th2) cells** which is important as a **B-cell** growth factor but which also down-regulates **T-helper cell type I (Th1)** immune responses. |

| Interleukin (IL)-12 | A **cytokine** made by **antigen-presenting cells (APCs)** that makes virgin **T cells** become **T-helper cell type I (Th1) cells**. |

| Intractable diarrhea | Diarrhea that does not improve under any medical management. |

| Invariant chain | A molecule present in **class II major histocompatibility complex (MHC) molecules** that prevents self peptides binding to the groove of the MHC molecule as it is being made in the endoplasmic reticulum (ER). |

| Isotope switching | The process by which **B cells** change the **heavy chain** they make from **immunoglobulin (Ig)M** to IgG, IgA, or IgE, while retaining the same **variable (V) region**. |

J

| J chain | A molecule that joins polymeric **antibody** molecules together. For example, **immunoglobulin (Ig)A**, as present in secretions, is a dimer made up of two IgA molecules joined by a J chain. |

L

| Lamina propria (LP) | The loose area of connective tissue in the gut below the **epithelium**, and above the muscularis mucosa. |

| Langerhans cells | Specialized **dendritic cells** in the skin. |

| Lymphocyte function-associated antigen (LFA)1 | A molecule on **T cells** that binds to **intercellular cell adhesion molecule (ICAM)1** on **antigen-presenting cells (APCs)** and **endothelial** cells in blood vessels. |

Light chain	Part of the **antibody** molecule linked to the **heavy chain**. Antibody molecules have two light chains and two heavy chains.
Lipopolysaccharide (LPS)	A cell wall component of **Gram**-negative bacteria. Many cells in the body have cell surface receptors for **LPS**, called **Toll-like receptor 4 (TLR)**.
Lymphadenopathy	Swelling of the **lymph nodes**.
Lymphoepithelium	Any **epithelium** that contains **lymphocytes**.
Lymphoma	A malignant proliferation of **lymphocytes**, occurring mainly within the reticuloendothelial system, eg, **lymph nodes**.
Lymphopenia	An abnormally low concentration of lymphocytes within the blood.
Lymphoreticular system	The cells and tissues comprising the immune system (eg, the **lymph nodes** and **spleen**).
Lysozyme	An anti-bacterial molecule found in Paneth cells.

M

M cells	The specialized **epithelial** cells in **follicle-associated epithelium (FAE)** that phagocytosis **antigens** and particles from the gut and transport them into the **follicles**.
Macrophage	Phagocytic cells in tissues derived from blood **monocytes**.
Major histocompatibility complex (MHC)	A region of DNA, found on chromosome 6 in humans, that contains a large number of genes involved in the immune system.
Mast cell	A long-lived, bone marrow-derived cell that is present throughout the connective tissue of the gut, skin, and airway. It contains granules that are released following cross-linking of **immunoglobulin (Ig)E** bound to the mast cell surface, and that cause **type I hypersensitivity**.

Medulla	The central area of the **thymus** containing newly differentiated mature **T cells**, or the inner part of a **lymph node**.
Memory cell	A **B cell** or **T cell** that has previously encountered a particular **antigen** and that is often long-lived.
Metaplastic	In the context of the gut, the appearance of **epithelium** from another site, such as stomach epithelium appearing in the duodenum.
β2-Microglobulin	A molecule present on **class I major histocompatibility complex (MHC) molecules**. It is identical in all individuals.
Mucosa	The soft layer that lines the bowel above the muscularis mucosa and which contains the **epithelium** and **lamina propria (LP)**.
Mucosal addressin cell adhesion molecule (MAdCAM) 1	The molecule present on blood vessels in the gut wall that is the receptor for **α4β7 integrin** and controls the migration of cells into the **lamina propria (LP)**.
Multinucleate giant cell	Cell resulting from the fusion of several **macrophages**, characteristically (but not exclusively) associated with **granulomas**.
Myeloma	A malignant tumor of **plasma cells**.

N

N-region insertions	During **T cell** and **B cell receptor** rearrangement, the insertion of random nucleotides into the **variable (V) region**. This increases diversity.
Natural killer cells	A small cell population in blood that has the capacity to recognize and kill tumor cells and virally infected cells.
Negative selection	The elimination, mostly in the **thymus**, of **T cells** with receptors that bind self antigens. Also known as **clonal deletion**.
Neoplasm	A benign or malignant tumor.
Neuropathy	Inflammation of the nerves.

NOD2	A protein found inside cells that binds muramyl dipeptide (a component of the **Gram**-positive bacterial cell wall). Signaling through NOD2 tends to induce proinflammatory cytokine production. Also known as **CARD15**. It is mutated in about 15% of Crohn's patients.
Nodular lymphoid hyperplasia	An increase in the size of the **Peyer's patches (PPs)** or colonic lymphoid **follicles** in the **mucosa**, particularly common in children.

O

Oral tolerance	An immunologic phenomenon whereby feeding **antigen** renders an animal unresponsive to subsequent systemic immunization with the same antigen.
Otitis media	Infection of the middle ear.

P

Paneth cell	Specialized **epithelial** cells found at the base of the crypts in the small intestine that contain **defensins** and **lysozyme**. In inflammation, Paneth cell **metaplasia** occurs in the colon.
Pathogen	An infectious microbe or parasite that causes disease.
Petechiae	Small areas of bleeding (eg, within a **mucosal** surface).
Peyer's patch (PP)	The organized lymphoid tissue of the small intestine; predominant in the ileum.
Plasma cell	A differentiated **B cell** that makes large amounts of **antibody**.
Polymorphic	Genes that vary greatly between individuals. The human leukocyte antigen (HLA) system, synonymous with **major histocompatibility complex (MHC)**, is highly polymorphic. Transplants between unrelated individuals fail largely because MHC

molecules on grafts are recognized as foreign by the host immune system.

Polymyalgia Inflammation of the muscles.

Postenteritis syndrome Diarrhea that continues after an infection, especially in children, and is believed to be due to damage to the small bowel **mucosa**.

Proctitis Inflammation of the rectum.

Pyoderma gangrenosum Severe skin **ulcers** that may occur in patients with inflammatory bowel disease (IBD).

Pyrexia Fever.

S

Scleroderma An autoimmune disease characterized by chronic inflammation and progressive thickening of the skin.

Sclerosing cholangitis Inflammation and stricturing or destruction of bile ducts within or outside the liver.

Secretory component (polymeric immunoglobulin [Ig] receptor) A molecule made by **epithelial** cells, which, as the receptor for **J chain**, binds **IgA** and **IgM**. The epithelial cell then transports the IgA or IgM through its cytoplasm and secretes the **antibody** into the gut lumen.

Serotonin A product of **mast cells** that increases vascular permeability and induces contraction of smooth muscle cells. Also known as **5-hydroxytryptamine**.

Serum sickness A disease caused by the formation of immune complexes in the blood. These are then deposited in the joints and kidneys, where they fix **complement** and cause tissue damage.

Sigmoid colon The section of the distal colon between the rectum and the descending colon.

Somatic hypermutation The process that occurs in **germinal centers (GCs)** so that **antibody** molecules are made that progressively bind tighter and tighter to **antigens** during the course of the response.

Sprue	An older term used to designate flattening of the **mucosa**.
Steatorrhea	Stools that are pale and offensive due to increased fat content. Usually caused by either small bowel or exocrine pancreatic disease.

T

αβ T cell	A **T cell** bearing the αβ **T-cell receptor (TCR)**. These constitute the major T cell population in the body.
γδ T cell	A **T cell** that bears the γδ **T-cell receptor (TCR)**. These are uncommon in blood and lymphoid tissues, but are preferentially found in the gut **epithelium**.
T cell	A **lymphocyte** that comes from the **thymus** and is important in cell-mediated immunity (CMI).
T-cell receptor (TCR)	A molecule made up of two chains (αβ or γδ) which the **T cell** uses to recognize foreign peptides.
T-helper cell type I (Th1)	A particular type of **CD4 T cell** that secretes **interferon (IFN)**γ or **tumor necrosis factor (TNF)**α.
T-helper cell type II (Th2)	A particular type of **CD4 T cell** that secretes **interleukin (IL)-4, IL-5, IL-10**, and IL-13, and is important in allergic responses.
Thoracic duct	The vessel into which **lymph** from the gut drains. The **thoracic duct** enters the vena cava to deliver **lymphocytes** from the **lymph nodes** and tissues back into the blood.
Thymus	The tissue in the chest where **T cells** develop.
Toll-like receptors (TLRs)	A family of molecules that is present on many cell types. TLRs recognize bacterial products. Generally, binding of bacterial products to TLRs activates inflammatory pathways, such as the production of **tumor necrosis factor (TNF)**α. TLR2 recognizes peptidoglycan from **Gram**-positive bacteria, TLR4 recognizes **lipopolysaccharide (LPS)**, and TLR9 recognizes bacteria DNA.

Toxic megacolon	A very serious complication of ulcerative colitis (UC) in which the colon becomes very large and may perforate.
Transporter of antigenic peptides (TAP)	The molecules inside a cell that transport small peptides from the cytoplasm of the cell into the endoplasmic reticulum (ER) where the peptides can bind to **class I major histocompatibility complex (MHC) molecules**. It is the method by which the immune system is made aware of self and non-self **antigens** in the cytoplasm of cells.
Travelers' enteritis	Inflammation of the intestine, usually infectious in nature.
Trophozoite	The free-living form of a protozoan parasite.
Tumor necrosis factor (TNF)α	A molecule made by **T-helper cell type I (Th1) cells** and activated **macrophages** that can kill cells and increase adhesion molecules on **endothelial** cells, and is important in the formation of **granulomas**.
Type I hypersensitivity	The very rapid response in the skin or gut that occurs in minutes when an **antigen** binds to **immunoglobulin (Ig)E** on a **mast cell** and the mast cell releases its granules. Also known as **immediate hypersensitivity**.
Type II hypersensitivity	The response which occurs when **antibodies** are made against surface molecules on host cells.
Type III hypersensitivity	The **hypersensitivity** response due to the formation of immune complexes in blood or tissues (see **serum sickness, Arthus reaction**).
Type IV hypersensitivity	The slow inflammatory response that occurs when a memory **T cell** recognizes its **antigen** in the skin or other tissues and secretes **cytokines**, which cause **macrophages** to move from the blood into the tissue. Also known as **delayed-type hypersensitivity**.

U

Ulcer	Loss of an **epithelial** surface, as occurs within the bowel in inflammatory bowel disease (IBD).

| Urticaria | An itchy skin rash resulting from the release of **histamine** by **mast cells**. |
| Uveitis | Inflammation of the uveal tract of the eye (ie, the choroid and iris). |

V

Variable (V) region	The part of the **antibody** molecule that is very variable between different antibody molecules in the same individual and allows **B cells** to recognize millions of different **antigens**.
Vascular adhesion molecule	A molecule present on the surface of cells lining the blood vessels, which binds to molecules present on the surface of white blood cells. Examples include **intracellular cell adhesion molecule (ICAM)1**, vascular cell adhesion molecule 1, **mucosal addressin cell adhesion molecule (MAdCAM)1**, and **E-selectin**. Vascular adhesion molecule expression is increased by pro-inflammatory **cytokines**.
Vasculitis	Inflammation of the blood vessels.
Villus	The finger-like projections in the small intestine that increase the surface area available for food absorption.

Index

Page numbers in **bold** refer to figures: page numbers in *italics* refer to boxed material (b) and tables (t).

---

type I hypersensitivity 42
thymus, T-cell development 10–11
tissue destruction, inflammation 49
Toll-like receptors, innate immunity 1–2
Toxoplasma gondii infections,
immunocompromised patients 39
transforming growth factor-β (TGF-β), mastocytosis 118
traveler's diarrhea, *Campylobacter* enterocolitis 61
trichuriasis 139–40
tropical sprue 140–1
tumor necrosis factor-α (TNF-α)
    inflammation 47,48
    mastocytosis 118
    neonatal necrotizing enterocolitis 119
    production
        CD4 T-cells 17,**19**
        macrophages 2
        T-helper type I cells 20
    type I hypersensitivity 41
Turcot syndrome, colorectal carcinoma 66
type I hypersensitivity *see* hypersensitivity
type II hypersensitivity 43–4
type III hypersensitivity 44–5

U

ulcerative colitis 142–6
    age of onset 142
    clinical features 142
    diagnosis 143
    disease association 142
    epidemiology 142
    extraintestinal manifestations 142–3
    genetics 142
    histology **144–5**
    immunopathogenesis 143,**146**,146
    immunopathology 143,**144–5**
    lesion location 142
    surgery, pouchitis 127–8
    treatment 146

type II hypersensitivity 44
type III hypersensitivity 45
urticaria pigmentosa, mastocytosis 117
uveitis
    Crohn's disease 88
    ulcerative colitis 142

V

vacuolating toxin A (VacA),
Helicobacter-associated gastritis 110
variable regions, antibodies 6
vasculitis 147–9
    anti-inflammatory therapy 149
    Behçet's disease 147
    Churg–Strauss vasculitis 147
    Henoch–Schönlein disease 147
    histology 147
    immunopathology **148**
    Kawasaki disease 147
    polyarteritis nodosum 147
    Sjögren's syndrome 147
    Wegener's granulomatosis 147
villus, columnar epithelium 28
viral infections, CD8 T-cells 16
vitamin B_{12} deficiency, pernicious anemia 121

W

Wegener's granulomatosis, vasculitis 147
Whipple's disease 149–51
    antibiotic therapy 151
    histology **150**
    Th1 response 151

Y

Yersinia enterocolitis 151–3
    antibiotic therapy 153
    Crohn's disease *vs.* 153
    histology **152**
    microfold cells 153